GLENVIEW PUBLIC LIBRARY

3 1170 00533 9134

THE HEMP COOKBOOK

D1473475

THE HEMP COOKBOOK

FROM SEED TO SHINING SEED

TODD DALOTTO

Healing Arts Press
Rochester, Vermont

641.6353
DAL

Glenview Public Library
1930 Glenview Road
Glenview, Illinois

Healing Arts Press
One Park Street
Rochester, Vermont 05767
www.InnerTraditions.com

Healing Arts Press is a division of Inner Traditions International

Copyright © 2000 by Todd Dalotto

All rights reserved. No part of this book may be reproduced or utilized in any form or by any means, electronic or mechanical, including photocopying, recording, or by any information storage and retrieval system, without permission in writing from the publisher.

Note to the reader: This book is intended as an informational guide. The remedies, approaches, and techniques described herein are meant to supplement, and not to be a substitute for, professional medical care or treatment. They should not be used to treat a serious ailment without prior consultation with a qualified health care professional.

LIBRARY OF CONGRESS CATALOGING-IN-PUBLICATION DATA
Dalotto, Todd 1970-
    The hemp cookbook : from seed to shining seed / Todd Dalotto.
       p.   cm.
    Includes bibliographical references (p.).
    ISBN 0-89281-787-9 (alk. paper)
    1. Cookery (Hemp) 2. Hemp. I. Title.
TX814.5.H45 D35 1999
641.6'353—dc21
                                       99-40750

Printed and bound in Canada

10 9 8 7 6 5 4 3 2 1

Text design and layout by Kristin Camp
This book was typeset in Clearface with Craw Modern as the display typeface

JUN 20 2000

As we do before meals, let us give thanks:
To the cannabis plant.
Born of the earth;
offering its essence and entirety for healing on all levels;
praises to the plant that transforms the energies of pain,
    fear, and destruction
into healing, strength, and creation.

We—
children of the earth,
healers,
cultivators—

are here to resonate with your healing energies for the
    good of all life.

We are the root
grounded and firmly connected to the earth.

We are the stalk;
we rise up and emanate our strength.

We are the leaves,
beauty and gentleness.

We are the flowers,
freely sharing our healing gifts.

We are the seeds,
the children
and nourishment for all life.

Contents

Part 2: Hempseed in a Garden of Healing Foods

Part 3: Further Tales of Hempseed

Introduction

MY LIFE AS A HEMPSTER began in the fifth grade. The assignment was to write a factual report; the teacher left the topic open. Naturally I chose the most deviant subject in the library—marijuana. While researching the topic, I stumbled upon some rather unexpected historical facts. Different strains of the same plant, *Cannabis sativa,* had long been used to make rope, paper, and cloth.

The nature of my interest shifted swiftly from sheerly mischievous to genuinely inquisitive. I cited historical evidence such as: the founding fathers of the United States were hemp farmers; the first American flag was made of hemp; the original draft of the U.S. Constitution was written on hemp paper; and that hemp was a major agricultural product in America until the 1940s.

To my dismay, the first school assignment that I was truly proud of received a

"D" grade. There it was in red ink, "Well written, but the assignment was to write a *factual* report." My life was transformed forever and my purpose was becoming apparent. I knew there must be a world of obscured truths and it was my job to challenge the dominant paradigm by disclosing them. That sounds awfully heavy for a ten year old, but that's the way I understand it now.

Meanwhile, I was discovering my love for cooking. My mother worked two jobs and couldn't make dinner for us every night. My sister and I often fended for ourselves with the cupboard full of macaroni and cheese. Refusing to give in to the monotony of mac and cheese every night, I began my self-taught endeavor of creative cooking.

My father, a second generation Italian American, helped me to discover the high connection between gardening and cooking. As a youngster I helped him bring tomatoes, eggplant, basil, and herbs from the garden to the kitchen, then to the dinner table. Ah, the appreciation of eating homegrown food!

As a young adult, my lifestyle became centered around living in harmony with the natural world and protecting Mother Earth from the modern world that threatens her. My life as an activist became tiring. I worked hard to fight the huge collective corporate monster that is rapidly devouring all that is good on this planet.

What seemed to be missing from my activism was a viable solution that everyone could live with. In the early 1990s, with the help of Jack Herer's book, *The Emperor Wears No Clothes* (see appendix 2, "Suggested Reading"), I was awakened to the idea that many of the world's biggest ecological problems could be solved by centering industry around the use of Earth's most amazing renewable natural resource—cannabis hemp.

I also learned that hempseed is one of the most nutritionally complete foods on the planet. Not only does it contain protein, it contains an abundant supply of important nutrients (essential fatty acids) that are nearly missing from common diets. If used as a staple food and nutritional supplement, hempseed can help heal or even prevent many of the most common degenerative diseases.

My greatest focus as an activist had been to encourage people to change their lifestyles by living simply, not using toxins, and living in harmony with nature. With commonsense, hemp-based industries, the change could occur without much effort. This insight blew my mind. I realized that every person on this planet could participate in the transformation without even stepping out of their current roles in life.

I set out on a vision quest to discover how I could best participate in this healing revolution. The vision was clear: to synchronize my talents as a healing food-crafter, an activist, and an Earth caretaker. It all came together in the form of a business I started in Eugene, Oregon, in 1994 called Hungry Bear Hemp Foods.

I successfully ran Hungry Bear Hemp Foods for three years, producing some of the first hemp food products on the market: candy bars called *Seedy Sweeties*, flours, butter, shakes, smoothies, and milk. The national media attention I received helped to spread the word about hempseed's incredible value as a nutritious food.

You are holding in your hands the next stage of the vision. This is the culmination of the past six years of my healing and culinary relationship with the greatest seed on Earth. My hopes are to inspire you, as I have been inspired, to improve the health of the planet and each other by making the best use of the hempseed.

"Hempseed Overview" will take you through the history of the hempseed and its cultivation, handling, and other uses. Once you've whet your appetite with "The Healing and Nutritive Qualities of Hempseed," "Hemp Food-Crafting 101" will give you a basic course on the transformation of hempseed into basic products such as oil, flour, and butter. With this knowledge you can easily follow the recipes and experiment with your own hempseed culinary creations.

We'll celebrate the synthesis of cultivation and culinary arts in "Hempseed in a Garden of Healing Foods"—where you'll find soups, entrées, salads, dips, breads, desserts . . . and more. Not only does hempseed polish the glow of *our* health, it helps the songbirds sing and the cows jump over the moon—read "Food for Feathers, Fins, and Four Legs."

Be aware that recent studies and incidents have shown that the consumption of whole hempseed may result in a positive urine test of THC metabolites. Get informed and protect your rights by reading "Free To Pee THC."

Finally, the "Hemp Food Resource Directory" (appendix 1) can help you connect with those involved with hempseed foods. You can also enhance your own hemp food journeys by looking into "Suggested Reading" (appendix 2).

PART 1

Hempseed
Basics

Hempseed Overview

CANNABIS IS THE PLANT GENUS in the family Cannabinaceae, of the order Urticales (nettle). Due to morphological and anatomical similarities, it was once classified in the mulberry family (Moroaceae). Many modern botanists classify the *Cannabis* genus as having only one species, *sativa*, consisting of the varieties *C. sativa* var. *indica* (Indian hemp), *C. sativa* var. *ruderalis* (wild hemp), and *C. sativa* var. *vulgaris* (cultivated hemp).[1] These variety names have always been alternative species names in the *Cannabis* genus. This confusion should not be a factor in this book, though, because most food and fiber species are *C. sativa*.

Hempseed is technically an achene, an indehiscent fruit that is small and dry and usually contains an oily germ. Sunflower seeds are familiar examples of achenes. The hard hulls of achenes usually have no significant nutritional value and are often removed before consumption. Although hempseed hulls are among the easiest of achenes for us to chew and digest, hulled hempseed is highly desired, and is now beginning to take shape as a staple form of hemp food.

I know of no other plant that offers so much to aid in the survival of all life on this planet. *Cannabis sativa* is living proof of how forgiving Mother Nature is to a species that has caused her so much destruction. Despite our habits of consuming enormous amounts of precious resources, producing toxic and radioactive materials, and engaging in countless acts of hatred and war, *Cannabis sativa* has evolved to offer its fiber as a healthy, sustainable alternative to logging, cotton growing, and synthetic-fiber production. Its roots cleanse the soil and prevent erosion; its leaves replace nutrients in the soil; its seeds provide a cleaner-burning fuel than any petrochemical; and its flower eases our suffering, reduces our stress, and inspires our creativity.

I've written this book to share with you what I know about the ways we can use the seed of this splendiferous plant for the healing of our bodies, our spirits, and our home (planet). For further research into all the numerous nonfood uses of the cannabis plant, check out appendix 2, "Suggested Reading."

Cannabis didn't just pop out of the sky in recent times to save the world. There must have been some sort of intelligence that created this plant long before human civilization evolved, knowing that it would someday come in handy.

Humans caught on to the uses of the cannabis plant about ten thousand years ago. Across Eurasia ancient peoples used the fiber for textiles and pottery. Evidence of hemp cultivation in Egypt dates back to 4000 B.C. Indeed, hemp may have been human civilization's first agricultural crop.

The first recorded use of hempseed as food was in the first-century A.D. writings of the Greek physician, botanist, and philosopher Dioscorides. Galen, another physician-philosopher, recorded that in second-century Greece and Rome some people enjoyed eating fried hempseed with their dessert.[2] (See "Hempseed Medicine" on page 30 for more.)

The Polish and Lithuanian people make a hempseed soup called *semieniatka*. They traditionally served it to honor visiting spirits of their dead relatives.[3] The

THE USES OF HEMP

Plant Part	Yield per Acre	Ecological Benefits	Craft Applications	Industrial End Products
Root	8–9% of total plant mass	Deep taproot breaks up soil; weed suppression; adds organic mass	Medicinal extracts and preparations	No big demand currently
Stalk: bast (long outer fibers); hurds (short inner fiber); woody fibers	Stalk: 3–6 short tons; fiber: 1–2 short tons	Alternative to the world's most polluting industries; nontoxic farming and processing	Jewelry, weaving, knotting, carving, beads, pipe stems, paper . . .	Paper, building materials, cellulose plastics, methanol, clothing, rope . . .
Leaves	25% of total plant mass	Green manure; cleanses the air	Foods, pigments, visual arts	Pigments, animal bedding, compost
Flowers (low THC)	1,200 lbs.	Produces insect repellent	Aromatherapy, topical medicinal applications, food	Essential oils, fragrances, sunscreen, flavorings
Seeds	600–900 lbs.	Alternative to petrochemical products proliferation	Food, gardening	Highly nutritious oil, high-protein flour, dehulled seed meat, various foods, body care, industrial lubricants, diesel fuel . . .

Ukrainian and Latvian people make a similar offering on the Day of Three Kings.[4] Hempseed has long been a staple in Russia, too, where it's ground into butter and eaten as a gruel.

European monks were once required to eat hempseed in soups, gruel, or porridges three meals a day.[5] In southern Africa mothers of the Sotho tribe served the ground seeds with bread or mealie-pap to children during weaning as recently as the 1950s.[6] (Mealie-pap is a liquefied meal made from fresh corn.)

Until recently the main consumers of hempseed in North America have been commercially raised pigeons and canaries (see "Food for Feathers, Fins, and Four Legs"). Therefore, most of the imported and cultivated hempseed has been grown, handled, and traded using the standards of the birdseed industry. Unfortunately for the birds, this standard falls far below any criterion that would apply to any human food.

When the hemp food industry began in the early 1990s the quality of hempseed available was often not much better than birdseed. Responsible hemp food-crafters had to take precautionary measures such as lab testing or importing their own seed to ensure quality.

With every batch of seed I acquired, I sent a sample to an analytical lab for the following tests:

- *Peroxide value and free fatty acids*—these tests together determine how much oxidation has occurred. A peroxide value under 7 is acceptable. Values over 10 are usually perceivably rancid.
- *Bromide residues*—this test will detect the residue of common fumigants that may have been used in the warehouse or in shipment.
- *Pesticide residues*—tests any number of the most common pesticides.

Each set of these tests cost me up to $200, but I felt it worthwhile to ensure good products. The tests invariably resulted in no detectable pesticides or bromides and a safe peroxide value. Before investing in these tests, I performed a taste test myself, and then sought out a friend whose parrot loved hempseed. The parrot's palate was so sensitive that she rejected any seed that wasn't fresh enough. I found this to be a reliable test.

Having seed mechanically cleaned is extremely important, especially if you are pressing oil, as a single rock can ruin a $100,000 oil press. When my production was light, I cleaned my seed on demand using the wet method described in "Hemp Food-Crafting 101." When my production increased and my product line expanded, I had each batch of seed mechanically cleaned.

Mechanical seed cleaning involves either using a simple screen separator alone, or putting the seed through a series of processes. The screen separator shakes the seed through a series of screens, each with different-sized holes. This separates hempseed from anything else of different size. Even after a good run through a screen separator, though, I found pebbles the size of hempseed, so I used a second method: sending the seeds through a cylindrical tumbler that separated objects of different weights. More sophisticated tumblers are magnetized to remove any metal objects.

As the hemp food industry matures, our standards increase. Today, there is hempseed growing on almost every continent. The suppliers are more accessible, reliable, and accountable. These companies are often involved in the farming, processing, and marketing of their product.

STERILIZATION NATION

The United States is the only nation in the world that requires hempseed to be rendered "incapable of germination" upon importation. This restriction is a compromise reached during prohibition, when the birdseed lobby pleaded with Congress to allow canaries to keep eating their favorite food.

The method most commonly used is steam sterilization. This is performed by licensed facilities not only on hempseed, but also on other restricted seeds. Niger seed, for instance, is also a favorite of birds, but the species would be invasive if allowed to propagate. As we know, propagation of cannabis would be a very good thing.

The process involves placing the seeds in a chamber. Steam is injected, and the temperature is brought to at least 212°F (100°C) for fifteen minutes. At this temperature the enzymes needed for germination are killed.

Government regulations allow up to 2 percent of a sample of seeds to germinate. If more than 2 percent sprouts, then back to the gas chamber they go. Samples are not tested routinely.

A common misconception about hempseed sterilization is that it is performed to destroy THC. The opposite is actually true. Most of the THC in cannabis flowers is found in the form of THC-COOH (THC acid). This form of THC will not get you high, not even in large quantities. THC acid must be heated to around 200°F (93°C) in order for decarboxylation to occur, converting it to Δ-9 THC, the bioavailable form of THC. Depending on how well the seed was cleaned, it will contain some trace residues (measured in nanograms, or millionths of a gram) of THC-COOH. When hempseed is steam sterilized, then, its minute quantity of THC acid is converted to active THC—but you'd need to consume several hundred pounds of seed in a fifteen-minute period even to catch a buzz.

The exact impact that sterilization has upon hempseed's nutritional value has not been verified. Comparative nutritional analyses of sterilized and nonsterilized seed don't indicate much of a difference. However, even though a lab test shows no difference in the seed's *quantity* of protein, that protein may in fact become denatured and insoluble after undergoing such heat. What has been observed is a shorter shelf life and compromised taste. I personally can tell the difference by the way my body feels. If the U.S. government insists on continuing its hempseed-killing program, further tests should be performed to verify the effects of sterilization.

In 1994 Safari Seeds and Organics imported into the United States the first nonsterilized hempseed since before prohibition—legally! You see, regulations don't specify that hempseed must be steam sterilized, just that they be "incapable of germination." Safari Seeds grew a crop of hempseed in Chile, pressed it for oil, then shipped both the oil and pressed seed into the United States. Since neither the oil nor the pressed seed was capable of germination, both cleared customs with no problems.

HempNut, Inc., is taking a similar approach with its hulled hempseed product, HempNut.

The benefit of these approaches is that folks in the United States have a way to consume nonsterilized hempseed foods. The drawback is that we are still denied locally grown and produced hemp foods.

QUALITY ASSURANCES

Now that the major producers of hempseed for human consumption are gaining control over the trade and cultivation of their main ingredient, a higher standard of quality is being established.

The Hemp Food Association (see appendix 1, "Hemp Food Resource Directory") has been formed to set a standard of quality for hemp foods, as well as to establish a line of defense from the attacks that have been directed at the hemp food industry by groups such as the drug-testing industry, law enforcement, and federal government. It also creates opportunities for hemp food producers and experts to create mutually supportive relations.

Membership in the HFA requires agreeing to a pledge of quality that includes the following promises:

- To use only food-grade hempseed for human foods
- To avoid hempseed known to contain, or grown in areas known to have, excessive concentrations of radioactive elements or heavy metals
- To follow currently accepted good manufacturing processes
- To strive to develop written plans for good manufacturing processes, hazard analysis, and critical control points
- To be licensed to produce human food by the appropriate government agencies

- To comply with applicable local, state, and federal laws as they relate to food processing, especially labeling
- To carry product liability insurance in an amount of not less than $500,000
- To keep detectable tetrahydrocannabinol levels below 50 milligrams per gram (50 ppm) in the finished product
- To routinely test finished products for their microbiological profile and peroxide value
- To make results of laboratory analyses available upon reasonable request
- To prepare Material Data Safety Sheets for products, as necessary
- To disclose on the package the percentage of hempseed content in finished product
- To ensure that all organic claims are in accordance with applicable laws
- To disseminate no erroneous information on hemp or hempseed
- To refrain from portraying a hempseed food as capable of intoxication, or as being made from high-THC cannabis
- To advise the HFA of misinformation printed or distributed on hempseed foods
- The most important issue of hempseed quality we must address is the protection of the precious oil from free-radical oxidation

The Healing and Nutritive Qualities of Hempseed

BORN FROM THE FLOWER OF THE CANNABIS PLANT is a seed bursting with vital energy that nourishes, heals, rebuilds, and fuels our living bodies. The nutrients that compose hempseed satisfy our dietary need for all four macronutrients. *Macronutrients* are those elements or groups of elements that are required for organisms to live healthfully. For plants the macronutrients are carbon, hydrogen, oxygen, nitrogen, phosphorus, and potassium. Those for humans are protein, fats, carbohydrates, and fiber.

Hempseed is packed (approximately 25 percent) with easily digestible proteins that contain all eight amino acids in favorable proportions. Another 30 or so percent of this precious seed is composed of fats. No need to be alarmed! As you read on about fatty acids, you will learn which types of fats can cause disease and

General Nutritional Analysis of Whole, Sterilized Hempseed*

Calories	503 Kcal
Protein (N x 6.25)	22.5%
Fat	30.0%
Carbohydrate	35.8%
Total dietary fiber	35.1%
Insoluble dietary fiber	32.1%
Soluble dietary fiber	3.0%
Ash	5.9%
Moisture	5.7%

Data provided by Don Wirtshafter.

*Note: Most likely some of these measurements were made on a dry weight basis and others with moisture content included. This is why the percentages add up to more than 100 percent.

which fats heal and nourish us. Rest assured that hempseed is a rich source of essential fatty acids, which are crucial to the healthy functioning of all the systems of our bodies.

Yet another 36 percent is carbohydrates. These are the most common organic compounds on Earth and include sugars, starches, cellulose, and chitin. They are synthesized in plants via photosynthesis. They serve our bodies as an immediate source of energy.

Dietary fiber composes much of the remainder of the mass of the seed. Fiber helps cleanse our digestive tract and aids in the absorption of other nutrients.

General Nutritional Analysis of Hempseed Flour (from nonsterilized pressed hempseed)

Crude protein	29.6%
Crude fat	4.9%
Carbohydrate	57.5%
Crude fiber	27.6%
Ash	8.0%
Moisture	8.8%
Dry matter	91.2%

Data from lab test commissioned by Hungry Bear Hemp Foods and Herbal Products and Development.

General Nutritional Analysis of HempNut™ *

Calories per 100 g	**567 Kcal**
Protein (N x 5.46)	**30.6%**
Fat	**47.2%**
Saturated fat	**5.2%**
Monounsaturated fat	**5.8%**
Polyunsaturated fat	**36.2%**
Carbohydrate	**10.9%**
Cholesterol	**0.0%**
Total dietary fiber	**6.0%**
Ash	**6.6%**
Moisture	**4.7%**

*HempNut is a hulled hempseed product.
Data provided by The Hemp Corporation.

Sugars Assay of HempNut™

Total sugars	**1.99%**
Fructose	**0.45%**
Glucose	**0.30%**
Sucrose	**1.24%**
Maltose	**<0.10%**
Lactose	**<0.10%**

Data provided by the Hemp Corporation.

PROTEIN

Hempseed protein builds our bodies as hemp
fiber builds the world we create.

If there is any way to make hemp a part of you, it is by consuming the high-protein seed. Proteins are the building materials for every cell in our bodies. They constitute 80 percent of our dry muscle weight, 70 percent of that of our skin, and 90 percent of that of our blood. Therefore, if high-protein hempseed is among your staple foods much of your body mass is literally composed of cannabis. Maybe someday the Hemp Industries Association (HIA) will certify those of us who are composed of at least 10 percent hemp!

Dietary proteins are organic molecules composed of one or more chains of approximately twenty different kinds of amino acids. They come in all shapes, sizes, and structures and perform a wide variety of vital functions. The sequence of and interactions among the amino acids that proteins are composed of determine their characteristics. Proteins are often classified as either *structural* (fibrous) or *biologically active* (globular). Structural proteins, such as collagen, keratin, and fibrinogen, are the main ingredients in bones, skin, hair, ligaments, feathers, and hooves. Biologically active proteins—mostly globulins—include hormones, hemoglobin, antibodies (immunoglobulins), and enzymes.

Our bodies break down the pro-

Amino Acid Composition of Hempseed (mg per gram)

Threonine	3.7
Valine	3.0
Methionine	2.6
Isoleucine	1.5
Leucine	7.1
Phenylalanine	3.5
Tryptophan	0.6
Lysine	4.3
*Histidine	2.5
*Arginine	18.8

Data provided by Don Wirtshafter.
*Essential only for growing children.

teins we eat back into amino acids. The aminos then go through a process called *protein synthesis* in which they are transformed into any of tens of thousands of proteins, depending on what the body needs at that moment. Aminos that were once part of a globular protein can be synthesized into a fibrous protein, and vice versa. This might occur if, for example, the body had muscle damage to repair.

The simple proteins (proteins composed purely of amino acids) found in cannabis seeds are composed of 65 percent globular edestin (the highest percentage in the plant kingdom[1]) and small quantities of albumin. Edestin is a type of globular protein that is not only very digestible but actually facilitates digestion as well. No surprise that edestin shares the same Greek root with the word *edible*.[2] Globulin edestin is a major component of the hempseed embryo, where it provides the enzymes needed for metabolic activity of the sprout.

What makes these globular proteins so special is that they are precursors to some of the most vital chemicals in the body: hormones, which regulate all our body processes; hemoglobin, which transports oxygen, carbon dioxide, and nitric oxide; enzymes, which catalyze and control biochemical reactions; and antibodies (immunoglobulins), which fend off invading bacteria, viruses, and toxins (antigens) as they enter the body.

When an antigen enters the body, it responds by producing immunoglobulins whose structure fits that of the antigen membrane, thereby deactivating it. Once

Nonessential Amino Acid Composition of Hempseed (mg per gram)

Phosphoserine	0.9
Aspartic acid + asparagine 19.8	
Glutamic acid + glutamine 34.8	
Serine	8.6
Proline	7.3
Glycine	9.7
Alanine	9.6
Cystine + cysteine	1.2
Cystathionine	0.9
Tyrosine	5.8
Ethanolamine	0.4

Data provided by Don Wirtshafter.

the invading cell is neutralized, other blood cells can finish it off. Immunoglobulins will then continue to circulate in the blood, saliva, lungs, and gastrointestinal tract (depending upon which type of antibody it is) for several weeks, providing continued resistance to the invading antigen.

It is true that the body can make globular proteins out of a pool of the right amino acids, even if they are structural in origin. However, it is much more efficient for the body to make globulins out of globular starting material. If the body has just enough of a supply of amino acids to prevent deficiency symptoms, it may not have enough globular protein on hand to produce antibodies if a virus should strike. This is why consuming foods high in globular protein is so vitally important. Therefore, consuming hempseed—which contain the highest percentage of globulin edestin in the plant kingdom—is a wise food choice.

The other significant protein contained in hempseed is called *albumin*. Albumin is water soluble and comprises the layer between the hull and embryo of the hempseed. When water soaks into the seed, the dissolved albumin protein becomes a ready source of energy for the awakened embryo. Albumin fuels the embryo as it breaks open the hull and finds the sun, for more energy.

Not only does hempseed contain these crucial types of proteins, but it also contains all eight essential amino acids in the same proportions that our bodies use them. *Essential amino acids* are those that must be included in our diets because our bodies cannot produce them. Hempseed also contains two amino acids that are essential for childhood growth but are less important in adult life. In addition, hempseed contains eleven other amino acids in varying quantities.

ESSENTIAL FATTY ACIDS

The health revolution will truly be upon us when we change the way we think about fats. Popular advertising has recently bestowed on us the erroneous concept that all fats are bad and should be avoided. Believing they are making a health-conscious decision, many fat-fearing folks have thus unknowingly eliminated from their diets one of our most precious nutrients: essential fatty acids (EFAs).

What *is* true in the media hype is that the way Americans consume fats increases the risk of heart attack, cholesterol buildup, high blood pressure, stroke, obesity, and various sorts of cardiovascular disease. What's left out of the hype is an explanation of exactly what is unhealthy about our fat consumption. Nearly all the food available to us is laden with saturated fats and highly refined oils. The only advantage of these fats is that they have a long shelf life. The main disadvantage is that large quantities of saturated fat in the diet can cause disease related to cholesterol buildup. In addition refined oils are void of nutritional value—and are, in many cases, actually toxic.

With the intention of selling you their no-fat, low-fat, or synthetic-fat food products, most manufacturers fail to mention that our bodies require quantities of certain types of fats to perform many vital functions. These are called *essential fatty acids* (EFAs).

Hempseed has the highest concentration of EFAs (80 percent of total oil volume) found in any food on the planet. There are two EFAs: alpha linolenic acid and linoleic acid. In hempseed, the two are found in the same ratio that many nutritionists agree is ideal for the human body's needs.

Alpha linolenic acid (LNA, 18:3w3) is an omega-3 superunsaturated essential fatty acid. As vital as it is to our health, it can only be found in significant quantities in such seeds as flax, chia, kukui, and blackcurrant. Small quantities can be found in canola (rapeseed) and pumpkin seed oils. Hempseed oil is composed of around 19 percent LNA. Only in the past two decades has LNA been given the attention and research that its counterpart, LA, has enjoyed. The exact amount needed in our diets remains unknown— and of course individual needs differ. Many experts agree upon 1 to 2 teaspoons per day, suggesting that 2 percent of our caloric intake be from LNA.

Symptoms of LNA deficiency include dry skin, growth retardation, weakness, impaired learning ability, poor motor coordination, behavioral changes, impaired vision, high blood pressure, sticky platelets, edema, mental deterioration, low metabolic rate, and immune dysfunction.

Linoleic acid (LA, 18:2w6) is an omega-6 polyunsaturated essential fatty acid. It is much more available in common foods than is LNA; the richest sources are nonhigholeic varieties of safflower and sunflower oils. Hempseed oil is composed of about 57 percent LA. Because LA is present in our bodies in much greater quantities than LNA, an optimum daily dosage would be around 2 to 6 teaspoons, or 3 to 6 percent of our caloric intake.

Symptoms of LA deficiency include skin eruptions (acne and eczemalike), loss of hair, poor blood circulation, behavioral disturbances, liver and kidney degeneration, gallbladder problems, prostatitis (inflammation of the prostate), muscle tremors, abnormal water loss through the skin, susceptibility to infections, impaired wound healing, male sterility, miscarriage, arthritis, cardiovascular disease, and growth retardation.

The deficiency symptoms described above are all reversible with adequate intake of EFAs. If ignored for a long time, they could develop into more serious degenerative conditions.

Hempseed oil also contains about 2 percent *gamma linolenic acid* (GLA, 18:3w6), which is an omega-6 polyunsaturated fatty acid. This is not considered an *essential* fatty acid because our bodies can produce it from LA—although many conditions of disease and nutritional deficiency can interfere with this process. GLA may thus be an EFA for individuals with blocking conditions such as old age, excess cholesterol, zinc deficiency, common viral infections, and diabetes; it can be essential for those who consume excess saturated fats, refined oils, fried foods, alcohol, and sugar.[3]

The benefits attributed to the ingestion of GLA are similar to those of the EFAs. GLA can also relieve symptoms of premenstrual syndrome and prevent Sjogren's syndrome (drying and atrophy of tear and salivary glands).[4]

Now that we know what happens when we *don't* consume EFAs, let's find out about what happens when we *do* consume them. This brings us to the marvelous topic of fatty acid metabolism.

Fat metabolism occurs mainly in the liver where, through various chemical changes, fats that are ingested or already present in the body are transformed into other substances that the body needs, burned as energy, or discarded as waste. Fatty acids, being carbon chains with hydrogen atoms attached all along, and an acid group at one end, are really just puzzles for our bodies to take apart, put together, lengthen, shorten, and manipulate as the enzymes see fit. Fatty acids are often converted by oxidation, desaturation (insertion of double bonds), and elongation of the chains.

EFAs are metabolized into prostaglandins—partially oxidized EFAs whose hormonelike properties regulate nearly every cellular function. EFAs, in both their original and their metabolized forms, are structural components of cell membranes, where they play an important role in the transfer of nutrients and wastes in and out of the cell. Here they also help transfer bioelectric currents from cell to cell. The ability of EFAs to hold oxygen in our cell membranes is an important contribution to a healthy immune system, for this oxygen acts as a barrier to invading viruses and bacteria.[5]

Inside the cell EFAs are important structural components in the membranes of many organelles. They also provide energy, regulatory function, immune protection, and structural material for cell division.

Over half the dry weight of our brains is lipids![6] Here fatty acids are used as structural components and for energy. Our brains require a minimum of 10 to 20 percent of our bodies caloric intake to function, and a diet rich in EFAs is important to healthy brain function. EFAs take part in synaptic activity, in the work of chemical receptor sites, as well as in the other important functions already described. Our brains prefer EFAs for these functions, but will use saturated fats if there are insufficient EFAs. If your brain is loaded with EFAs, then, you ought to be flattered when someone calls you a fathead! Likewise, a brain full of saturated fatty acids could appropriately be called a meathead.

Because EFAs are vital for brain development, the best time to start on an EFA-rich diet is in the womb. That means, of course, that the pregnant and lactating mother must consume EFAs in quantities that far exceed her personal needs if both she and her child are to benefit fully.

Whether they know it or not, athletes depend on EFAs for stamina and recovery from muscular fatigue. Muscle cramps related to exercise are largely caused by the buildup of lactic acid. EFAs aid in the conversion of lactic acid to water and carbon dioxide.

Our bodies use EFAs in a ratio of about 3:1 (LA:LNA). Many nutritionists recommend this ratio for our dietary intake of EFAs. It may or may not be a coincidence that hempseed oil contains EFAs in exactly this ratio. Unless hempseed oil is your sole source of fats, though, your diet probably favors LA derived from other vegetable oils. So to achieve the optimum balance in your diet, it may be wise to use other EFA-rich oils with different ratios along with hempseed oil. For example, if people who use safflower oil (LA rich) as their primary cooking oil also eat equal proportions of hempseed oil (3:1) and flax oil (1:3), they may achieve a 3:1 ratio in their overall EFA intake. Supreme 7 from Herbal Products and Development (see appendix 1) is a blend of seven nutritious oils (including hempseed) that results in a 1:1 ratio of EFAs.

Achieving that proper ratio is also important because recent research has pointed out that oils high in omega-6 fatty acids send a message to the genes to produce a cancer-promoting protein called *ras p21*. A proper ratio of omega-3 fatty acids will deactivate this protein.[7]

Although EFAs are a ready source of energy (calories), their primary roles are the important functions described above. Only after we have ingested ample EFAs for cellular functioning do our bodies even think of burning them for energy. Naturally, we wouldn't heat our homes with good lumber if we don't have enough to finish building the house! When we do have excess fatty acids to burn, our metabolic rates increase and our bodies burn fats and glucose faster, helping us burn excess fats stored as adipose tissue (body fat).

Our bodies' principal source of calories from fat is saturated fatty acids (SaFAs). SaFAs are abundant in animal foods (including eggs and dairy), and found in small quantities in vegetable oils. Hempseed oil is composed of about 8 percent saturated fat. When our energy needs are met, our bodies metabolize excess fatty acids into SaFAs for storage as adipose tissue.

COMPARATIVE FATTY ACID COMPOSITION
OF HEMPSEED AND OTHER OILS
(Figures for each fatty acid are % of total fat content)

Seed	Fat content (%)	ESSENTIAL FATTY ACID		OTHER IMPORTANT FATTY ACIDS			
		LNA omega-3	LA omega-6	GLA omega-6	Oleic acid	Stearic acid	Palmitic acid
Hemp	30–35	19–21	57–58	2	12	2	6
Flax	35	58	14	0	19	4	5
Evening primrose	17	0	72	9	11	2	6
Borage	*	4	38	19	*	*	*
Black currant	*	14.5	44	19	*	*	*
Walnut	60	5	51	0	28	5	11
Soybean	18	7	50	0	26	6	9
Olive	20	0	8	0	76	16	0
Canola	30	7	30	0	50	7	0
Safflower	60	0	75	0	13	12	0

*Data unavailable for these values.

Compiled from data provided by Udo Erasmus, Don Wirtshafter, and Kenneth Jones.

OTHER FATTY ACIDS IN HEMPSEED OIL

Fatty Acid Name	Structural Formula	% of Total Fatty Acids
Palmitoleic acid	16:1w7	6.1
Heptadecanoic acid	17:0	0.2
Arachiditic acid	20:0	0.5
Eicosenoic acid	20:1	0.3
Behenic acid	22:0	0.3
Erucic acid	22:1w9	0.2
Lignoceric acid	24:0	0.3
Nervonic acid	24:1	0.2

Data provided by Don Wirtshafter.

FATTY ACID BREAKDOWN OF HEMPNUT™*

Fatty Acid	Structural Formula	Quantity (%)	% of Total Fatty Acids
Total fat (per 100 grams 100 grams of HempNut)		47.2	100
Palmitic acid	16:0	3.44	7
Arachidic acid	20:0	0.28	0.6
Oleic acid	18:1w9	5.80	12
Linoleic acid (LA)	18:2w6	27.56	58
Alpha linolenic acid (LNA)	18:3w3	8.68	18
Stearic acid	18:0	1.46	3

*HempNut is a hulled hempseed product.
Data provided by The Hemp Corporation.

Foods that grow closer to the equator (tropical) have a higher quantity of SaFAs and less polyunsaturated fatty acids. The reverse is true for foods that grow closer to the poles (cold climates). The reason is that plants (and seeds) that must survive freezing temperatures produce fluids that remain liquid even below 32°F. (The same is true for cold-water fish and mammals.) Tropical plants produce oils that will remain stable in blazing-hot conditions.

SaFAs are often solid at room temperature, whereas polyunsaturated fatty acids are often liquid at below-freezing temperatures. When stored at 0°F (18°C) hempseed oil is a thick liquid with semisolids of coalesced SaFAs.

Currently, seed varieties are being thrown around from continent to continent and climate to climate. For example, instead of growing varieties that have been grown in North America for hundreds of years, Canadian farmers must obtain certified seed stock from Europe and start from scratch to breed varieties adapted to Canadian conditions. Once seeds are heirloomed in respective bioregions, we'll begin to benefit from the nutritional and medicinal differences among various strains and growing conditions.

We are currently rediscovering the marvelous attributes of the cannabis plant after its decades of receiving bad publicity. Likewise, we are realizing that the grim picture of fats is only a single scene in the sublime film on the life of lipids.

MICRONUTRIENTS

Micronutrients are substances, mainly vitamins and minerals, that are ingested or produced by our bodies in very small amounts necessary for functioning and growth. The best sources for micronutrients, in general, are fruits, green leafy veggies, and root veggies.

As much as I boast about hempseed being the most nutritionally complete natural food, I'll never say that you can subsist on it alone. In the coming pages, you'll be combining hempseed with a variety of foods that have their own unique nutritional merits. Given that hempseed will provide all the protein, carbohydrates, and EFAs you need, you'll naturally want to combine it with foods high in vitamins (green leafy veggies) and minerals (roots and sea veggies) for a nutritionally complete meal.

Ingesting an adequate supply of vitamins B_3, B_6, C, magnesium, and zinc is required for the conversion of EFAs into prostaglandins. As you'll see in the following tables, hempseed provides these nutrients in small quantities, so be sure to eat other foods rich in these nutrients to get the full benefits of EFAs.[8]

The vitamin assay table shows that just a handful of hempseed (about an ounce) provides many vitamins. Remember, of course, that the U.S. recommended daily allowance (RDA) suggests amounts necessary to prevent deficiency symptoms in the "average" person. Depending upon your individual needs, you may require more (most likely) or less than the suggested quantities.

The mineral quantities in the mineral assay table are not necessarily accurate for all sources of hempseed. Mineral content depends largely upon the mineral content of the soil the plant is grown in.

As you can see, the nutritional quantities of HempNut differ greatly from those of whole, sterilized hempseed.

VITAMIN ASSAY OF WHOLE, STERILIZED HEMPSEED

Vitamin	Quantity per Ounce of Hempseed	% U.S. RDA per Ounce of Hempseed
Carotene (precursor to vitamin A)	1,050.00 IU	21.0
Thiamine (vitamin B_1)	0.28 mg	23.0
Riboflavin (B_2)	0.34 mg	20.0
Pyridoxine (B_6)	0.09 mg	4.7
Niacin (B_3)	0.78 mg	3.9
Ascorbic acid (vitamin C)	0.44 mg	0.7
Calciferol (vitamin D)	< 3.10 IU	0.8
Tocopherol (vitamin E)	0.93 mg	3.1

Data adapted from the results of a nutritional and chemical analysis commissioned by Don Wirtshafter.

MINERAL ASSAY OF WHOLE, STERILIZED HEMPSEED

Element	Quantity (ppm)	Element	Quantity (ppm)	Element	Quantity (ppm)
Aluminum	54.00	Iodine	0.84	Silicon	13.80
Antimony	1.75	Iron	179.00	Silver	0.40
Arsenic	0.30	Lead	0.03	Sodium	22.00
Barium	6.48	Lithium	0.06	Strontium	7.33
Beryllium	0.04	Magnesium	6,059.00	Sulfur	2,394.00
Boron	9.50	Manganese	95.43	Thorium	8.12
Cadmium	0.28	Mercury	< 0.001	Tin	2.60
Calcium	1,680.00	Molybdenum	0.51	Titanium	1.78
Chromium	0.65	Nickel	5.00	Tungsten	1.84
Cobalt	0.53	Phosphorus	8,302.00	Vanadium	0.84
Copper	12.00	Platinum	9.23	Zinc	82.00
Germanium	2.67	Selenium	< 0.02	Zirconium	1.23

Data provided by Don Wirtshafter.

MINERAL ANALYSIS OF HEMPSEED FLOUR
(from nonsterilized pressed hempseed)

Mineral	Quantity
Boron	138.2 ppm
Copper	15 ppm
Iron	245 ppm
Manganese	95 ppm
Nitrogen	4.74%
Phosphorus	0.86%
Calcium	0.19%
Chloride	0%
Potassium	1.10%
Magnesium	0.84%
Sodium	0.20%
Sulfur	0.02%
Zinc	65 ppm

Data from lab tests commissioned by Hungry Bear Hemp Foods and Herbal Products and Development.

VITAMINS AND MINERAL ASSAY OF HEMPNUT™*

Nutrient	Quantity per Ounce of HempNut	% U.S. RDA per Ounce of HempNut
Beta-carotene (precursor to vitamin A)	1.16 IU	< 1.0
Thiamine (vitamin B$_1$)	0.4 mg	33.0
Riboflavin (B$_2$)	0.1 mg	6.0
Pyridoxine (B$_6$)	0.03 mg	1.5
Vitamin C	.29 mg	0.5
Vitamin D	660.5 IU	165.0
Vitamin E (dl-alpha tocopherol)	2.6 IU	8.7
Sodium	2.6 mg	<1.0
Calcium	21.5 mg	1.8
Iron	1.4 mg	7.7

*HempNut is a hulled hempseed product.
Data provided by The Hemp Corporation.

HEMPSEED MEDICINE

Long before modern science discovered the beneficial biochemical actions of hempseed's nutrients, the medicinal properties of hempseed were widely used in herbal medicine of both the East and West. To avoid confusion, in this section I'll cover the medicinal properties only of cannabis seeds, and not those of the THC-rich cannabis flowers and leaves.

The Greek physician Dioscorides (c. A.D. 40–90) recorded the use of hempseed for medicine as well as for food. In his work *De Materia Medica*, one of this millennium's most authoritative herbal and pharmacological information resources, he extols *Cannabis sativa* for its medicinal benefits and recognizes hemp's value for stout cordage. Dioscorides also had the honor of giving our favorite plant its botanical name.[9]

In the early centuries A.D. in Europe it was common to use hempseed oil (juice) as an analgesic for earaches and for expelling insects from inside the ear. Galen (A.D. 129–c.199), a famed physician and philosopher, believed that gout is caused by overindulgence. He found hempseed useful in the treatment of this painful disease. Pliny the Elder (A.D. 23-79) prescribed infusion of hemp root to ease the inflamed joints of gout sufferers.[10] Pliny was also the first known to prescribe hempseed as a laxative for farm animals.

Hempseed was also used quite extensively throughout Asia. Whether in the form of oil, decoction, powder, infusion, paste, or whole, it was a vital ingredient in many formulas.

The Chinese, whose common name for hempseed is *huo ma ren*,[11] offer the most extensive medicinal information on it, most notably in *Pen T'sao Kang Mu*, China's pharmacopoeia compiled by Li Shih Chen. In addition to the wealth of information and prescriptions packed into this work's large section on cannabis seed, there are numerous recipes, formulas, and preparation methods.

The Chinese attribute the following medicinal properties to cannabis seed: The seed's energetics are sweet and neutral. Meridians and organs affected are the spleen, stomach, colon, and large intestine. Properties are demulcent (soothes, protects, and nurtures intestinal membranes), nutritive (nourishing to the body), laxative (loosens, relaxes, or stimulates evacuation of the bowels), diuretic (increases blood flow through the kidneys and thus augments urination), anthelmintic (destroys and dispels parasites such as worms), and mild yin tonic.[12, 13]

According to the following bits and pieces of modern and ancient prescriptions found in Chinese medicinal texts, cannabis seed:

- Is a chi (life force) tonic
- Can be used to hasten childbirth where the delivery is troubled with complications, or overdue[14]
- Is indicated for postpartum recovery, for blood deficiency, and following febrile (fever) diseases
- Will alleviate retained placenta illness in mothers just beginning to suckle their infants[15]
- Increases the flow of mother's breast milk
- Is indicated in menstrual irregularities, constipation due to intestinal dryness, and wasting thirst[16]
- Is commonly prescribed to treat constipation, particularly in the elderly[17]
- Is indicated for dysentery[18]
- Is used as a treatment for obstinate vomiting[19]
- Is contraindicated for diarrhea[20]
- Is used as an assisting herb in formulas to treat ulcers and sores[21]
- Is helpful in reducing blood pressure
- Can break up long-standing problems with the blood flow[22]
- Will restore the blood, the pulse, and the veins and arteries[23]
- Improves the urinary tract and the passing of urine[24]
- Has the capacity to cure *zhong feng* (neurologic impairment due to stroke) and the problems of excess sweating that this brings on[25]
- Serve as a treatment for edema and its accumulation of diluted lymph[26]
- Promotes healthy hair and skin
- Accelerates hair growth[27]

Many of the preparation methods in *Pen T'sao Kang Mu* include high-heat cooking where the seed is often roasted, boiled, dehydrated, and pulverized. In *Planetary Herbology*, Michael Tierra suggests simmering 1 ounce of the pounded meal in 1 quart of water until the liquid reduces down to a pint. He recommends taking this in three doses throughout the day.

Today in China, cannabis seed oil in capsules is the most commonly prescribed remedy for constipation.

Hemp Food-Crafting 101

NOW THAT YOUR HEAD IS FULL OF GOOD REASONS to consume hempseed, we can shuffle into the kitchen and learn the first steps of hemp food-crafting. I'll describe here some hands-on basic techniques for transfiguring whole hempseed into its basic culinary forms: flour, milk, oil, and butter. These fundamentals will prime you for all the recipes that follow.

WASHED AND DRIED HEMPSEED

Now that you've read this far you should have a clear sense of the importance of using clean hempseed. Unless you know your seed to be food grade you should assume that it may contain rocks, dirt, and bird poop.

If you are also unaware of the freshness of your seed, you should conduct a simple taste test. If the seed doesn't have a fresh, nutty flavor, it may not be fresh enough to eat. If it tastes awful, burns your throat, or makes your cheeks cringe, it's probably rancid. Such seed should be composted so that not even the birds can get to it.

I know that all this talk of dirty, rancid seed may leave a bad taste in your mouth, but it should also prevent disgusting experiences with hempseed. I can't tell you how many times I've heard about people becoming totally turned off to hemp because an otherwise well-intentioned person fed them spoiled hemp food.

As the hemp food industry grows, the quality of seed improves. By the time the next edition of this book comes out, I hope to omit this section; by then we should have easy access to clean, locally grown, food-grade seed.

To wash seeds, simply place them in a large bowl. As you are filling the bowl with water, agitate the seeds by swishing them around with your hands. When the bowl is full, let it sit for 5 minutes. This is long enough for dirt and rocks to fall to the bottom. Seeds that have split hulls will fill with water and fall to the bottom as well. Split seeds are the result of steam or heat sterilization. Their germ has been exposed to oxygen and is probably rancid.

Now everything that you don't want is on the bottom, and all the good seed is floating on top. Using a hand strainer, skim the floating seeds off the top. Give the seeds one more good rinse through the colander and leave them to drain for a few minutes.

My favorite way to dry the seeds is to spread them out on a blanket of hemp fabric and leave them out in the summer sun. The birds appreciate this method, too! A food dehydrator will work as well, though.

If you can't wait all day for dry seeds, you can stir them in a wok over medium heat until dry. You can also spread them on a cookie sheet and place in an oven set to 200° to 250°F (93° to 121°C). Be careful not to roast the seeds (unless you want them roasted). If you hear seeds pop, then turn down the heat or remove the seed from it.

With some recipes you can start with wet or sprouted seeds. In this case, seed drying would be superfluous.

ROASTED HEMPSEED

Roasting is a process by which you cook food by exposing it to dry heat. When the hempseed is roasted, its "green," nutty flavor is transformed to a rich "brown" nutty flavor. The oil from the inside is liberated to the outside of the hull, and the seed becomes crunchier and easier to chew.

One of the first hemp food products to hit the market was roasted, seasoned hempseed packaged in 1-ounce plastic bags. This snack food is simple to produce and satisfies a wide range of taste buds. Since the oil has been cooked and liberated to the outside of the hull (exposed to heat, light, and oxygen), I would caution against eating anything but *freshly* roasted hempseed. A bag of roasted hempseed that you find at the store may have been on the shelf or in a warehouse for weeks or months. The seed may even taste good because the salt, seasonings, and spices override its rancid taste.

Given the above warning, you may wish to take that $2 you were going to spend on an ounce of roasted hempseed and invest it in the ingredients you'll need to fresh-roast at home yourself.

Begin with cleaned seed, either dry or wet (double the roasting time if you start with wet seed). In any of the following methods, your senses will tell you when the seed is roasted. Slightly browned seed that emanates an appealing nutty aroma is done to perfection.

Oven-Roasting

Preheat the oven to 250°F. Spread the seed over a cookie sheet no deeper than an inch. Bake for 30 minutes or until the popping sound slows.

Wok- or Skillet-Roasting

Heat a heavy steel hammered wok or a large iron skillet (unoiled) over a high flame. When the pan is thoroughly heated, reduce the heat to medium. Toss in hempseed and stir constantly for about 20 minutes.

Hot-Air Popper

To avoid electrical hazards, please don't use wet seed in this method. Using an ordinary hot-air popcorn popper, you can roast hempseed in ¼- to ½-cup batches. Just pour the seed in, turn the machine on, and keep your hand poised on the OFF button for the moment when your senses tell you it's ready. The seed doesn't pop out of the machine and into the bowl like popcorn does. Because the heat is so high, the window between "done" and "burned" is very slim; you must rely on your senses to flick the switch off at the precise moment. Depending on the wattage of your popper, this may take between 30 seconds and 3 minutes.

In this quicker and hotter process the germ of many of the popped seeds will puff like popcorn! My name for this is "potcorn."

I live off the grid, so it is a rarity for me to roast in this manner. However, I still have one popper for corn and another for hempseed. To keep your machine clean, it is a good idea to roast the seed bare and season it after you pour it out. Be aware that not all hot-air poppers work for hempseed. Choose one that is simple in design with a wide cylinder in which hot air circulates.

A properly roasted hempseed has a hull that is more brittle than a raw one. This makes it much easier for our teeth to do their job. The most common complaint about hempseed is that it is hard to chew. If you roast it before you throw it into any recipe, though, you'll reduce the chance of complaint.

To sample various seasonings for roasted hempseed, check out Seasoned Roasted Hempseed on page 51.

ROASTED HEMPSEED
MEAL AND FLOUR

Not only does roasting hempseed make the hull more brittle and easier to grind, but it evaporates some of the oil, thereby decreasing the oil content. These factors make for an easier job of flour and meal grinding (*flour* is a powder; *meal* is coarsely ground). Because of its strong flavor, even just a small proportion of roasted hempseed in multigrain flour will make the mix distinctively hempy. The process of flour grinding will be covered in more detail in the next section.

Roasted hempseed by itself can be easily ground into a coarse meal using a hand-cranked flour mill or food grinder. With most seed, you will end up with an oily yet crumbly meal. This increases the surface area and augments the rich roasted flavor. So potent is the flavor that I would classify it as a seasoning. Check out Roasted Hempseed Meal Seasoning on page 52 for some spicy ideas.

HEMPSEED FLOUR

When you see folks lined up at 6 A.M. waiting for the bakery to open, you get a sense of the value of freshly baked goods. The aroma of a day-old loaf of bread doesn't compare with that of a loaf coming right out of the oven. And once you understand the value of freshly baked, you can easily grasp the benefits of freshly ground flour.

Since whole hempseed has a high oil content (30 to 35 percent), grinding the seed alone will produce an oily paste instead of a dry flour. There are two ways to get around this. The simplest is to mix hempseed with dry grains and mill them together. With a ratio of 1 part hempseed to 2 or 3 parts dry grains, the total oil content falls below 15 percent, which will produce a powdery flour. Grains ground for flour typically have an oil content of less than 10 percent.

Whole wheat works great when mixed 2 parts wheat to 1 part hempseed. If you like to do the wheat-free thing, you ought to have a fine adventure experimenting with various grain and bean mixtures. My favorite combinations are hempseed mixed with:

- Oats, barley, millet
- Quinoa, amaranth, rice
- Lentil, soy

The other method is to mill hempseed cake or pressed seed (both explained in more detail below). Both of these by-products have a maximum oil content of 10 percent and can be ground on their own to produce 100 percent hempseed flour. At the time of this book's printing, neither the cake nor the pressed seed is available on the consumer level. So do some consumer activism and make sure your local grocery or co-op carries these vital ingredients.

Obviously, since you're using seed with a reduced oil content, you'll end up with fewer EFAs to benefit from. That's okay, though, because most ways in which you'll use the flour involve baking and cooking. The fewer polyunsaturated fatty acids that reach high temperatures, the more stable the recipe is against free-radical oxidation.

As the EFA content decreases, the percentage of protein increases! In recipes that include hempseed flour, I tend to bring the ratio back into balance by adding raw hempseed oil prior to serving. Protein isn't nearly as sensitive to heat as polyunsaturated fatty acids are.

If you have yet to discover the wondrous benefits of freshly grinding your own flour, I highly recommend you do so today. One you get started in it and find how easy and rewarding it is, you will wonder why you ever bought preground.

Your first step is to acquire a flour mill that suits your needs. There are a few hand-cranked models available, the most popular called the Corona. You may also find a food grinder in a thrift store that has a plate for flour grinding. And there are a few electric countertop models available, including the grain mill attachment for the Champion Juicer. Check out appendix 1 for distributors of mills.

Any of the above gadgets will make a quality flour suitable for most purposes. Most are screw-fed and have a pair of 3- or 4-inch grinding plates. Stone grinding surfaces (burrs) are preferred. The less expensive steel burrs will suffice, however, as long as they are kept sharp.

If you are a restaurateur or small-scale food producer, you will find quite a variety of machines to suit your needs. There are also flour mill attachments for mixers.

The more flour you consume, the more you will realize the importance of using an implement that can produce fine flour. When hempseed is coarsely ground or has coarse bits, the hull can have a slightly sharp feel. It took the destruction of an expensive hammer mill screen for me to learn about the abrasive qualities of the hempseed hull. In fact, I hope someone out there picks up on this idea to create hemp sandpaper and other abrasives!

Back to food . . .

Eating coarsely ground flour in moderation may be a beneficial intestinal cleanser, but a steady diet of it can irritate sensitive membranes, especially in the mouth and throat. I have memories of doing service at hemp food booths and munching down a coarse-flour cookie or two. Or three. Or four. When I lost count my raspy throat reminded me that I had had enough. I then felt soothing relief with a gargle of hempseed oil.

This is where hulled hempseed (described below) comes in. It is too oily to grind alone (unless you want a paste), so you will have to mix it with other grains.

If you don't use your freshly ground flour right away, keep it refrigerated in an airtight container. It will be stay good for about a week.

HEMPSEED OIL

Squeeze out the oil from hempseed and you'll enjoy the golden-green juice of life!

Of course, squeezing hempseed oil is not quite as simple as squeezing orange juice. Given its physical characteristics and ratio of oil to solid matter, hempseed must undergo thousands of times more pressure than you would exert to juice an orange. In fact, the more I think about it, the further juicing oranges seems from pressing hempseed oil. So let's leave the orange juice analogy behind or save it for a recipe later.

Hempseed produces a polyunsaturated oil that is highly reactive to light, heat, and oxygen; great care must therefore be taken with pressing, bottling, and storage.

A good batch of seed is the first step to achieving quality oil. Fresh seed is important. It should be less than a year old and stored properly in a clean, cool environment. There should be a high proportion (90 percent plus) of mature seed. Immature seed is paler green in color, is lightweight, will crush easily between your fingers, and does not contain a worthwhile quantity of oil. Good separating equipment should be able to remove immature seed.

Contrary to popular belief, bigger seed isn't better for pressing oil. Bigger seed contains a smaller percentage of oil and has a thicker hull. Therefore, your press will work harder (more heat) and yield less oil. In addition, when you separate your seed by size the screening for larger-size seed will allow larger pebbles to remain. It doesn't take many pebbles of any significant size to ruin a good oil press.

You are probably familiar with the term *cold-pressed*. This is an industry term that means an oil is pressed using mechanical means and comes out no warmer than 105°F (40°C). Which doesn't sound very *cold*, but we'll go along with the term for now. A little warmth actually makes the oil easier to extract. Therefore, efforts to chill the process would be self-defeating. Oil seeds are usually heated between 120° and 160°F (50° to 70°C) before pressing to increase yields.

At this time, freshly pressing your own hempseed oil (or any vegetable oil) is just a dream. The equipment required for pressing seed oil is quite sophisticated, expensive, and sizable. A more realistic vision would be a cooperatively owned oil press for your community. In this case, a community can support local agriculture, control quality, and provide the freshest, most nutritious seed oil possible. The environment also benefits because products aren't being transported to every corner of the world, and wasteful packaging can be minimized.

If an oil press has yet to sprout up in your community, you may have to go purchase or trade for some of this fine oil. Check out appendix 1 for sources. You may be able to either order direct or receive a wholesale catalog to pass on enthusiastically to your co-op or natural food store.

Here are a few important things to keep in mind while shopping for the best hempseed oil:

1. **Is the oil pressed from sterilized seed?** Nonsterilized hempseed has superior taste, shelf life, and nutrition. Although nonsterilized whole

seed is not allowed in the United States, nonsterilized hempseed *oil* is allowed (pressing oil renders the seed "incapable of germination," satisfying the regulations).

2. **What pressing method?** You're looking for oil labeled COLD-PRESSED, for the reasons described above. The only pressing method commonly bragged about on labels is EXPELLER-PRESSED. If the label isn't clear about the pressing method, it may have been solvent extracted (not good; see #4).

3. **Was the oil pressed and packaged in an oxygen-free environment?** As stated before, the oil's contact with oxygen will cause it to go rancid quickly. Quality oil producers press and bottle oil in an oxygen-free environment. In most cases they press and bottle in an enclosed system filled with nitrogen gas. Argon gas may also be used with nitrogen to make the gas heavier than oxygen. Manufacturers often have a trade name—such as Omegaflo—for their unique patented methods. If the first time the oil contacts oxygen is when you open it yourself, you've made a good choice!

4. **Was the oil processed with solvents or bleaching agents?** Although solvent-extracted and bleached vegetable oils look pretty and pure on the supermarket shelf, these processes severely hurt oil quality. Many oil producers use harsh solvents such as hexane to extract the remaining oil after the first cold-pressing to maximize yields. In my opinion solvent-extracted oil should be graded and sold as industrial grade, and not for human consumption.

HEMPSEED CAKE AND PRESSED SEED

When the oil is pressed out of hempseed, the remaining by-product is called hempseed cake or pressed seed, depending on the pressing method. Expeller presses grind the seed under enormous pressure and squeeze out a cake that is unrecognizable as the seed it once was. The pressed seed that comes out of a batch press (a pressing method that uses pressure without grinding) simply looks like squished seed.

Raw whole hempseed has an oil content of around 30 percent. Both of the above pressing methods extract about two-thirds of the seed's oil, leaving the pressed seed (cake) with an oil content of 10 percent.

Because of this reduced oil content, pressed seed (cake) is open to a world of food-crafting that isn't possible or stable given the polyunsaturated fatty acid content of raw whole hempseed, namely, high-temperature cooking.

HULLED HEMPSEED

From all the thousands of folks whom I've served hemp foods to over the years, the only consistent complaints I have heard about hempseed relate to the hull. It is abrasive, even when ground fine; it makes any type of grinding difficult; it gets stuck between the teeth; and it has no essential nutritional value.

Why does the plant even grow that dratted hull? Isn't the cannabis plant one of the Creator's most perfect creations? What's with this flaw?

Okay, back off. Don't forget it's that solid hull that seals in the precious oil, protecting it from oxygen, light, and little critters. Everything has its purpose.

Still, for many culinary purposes folks prefer to have the hull removed. Like licking the icing and leaving the cake. Folks in both Europe and the United States have thus been applying their ingenuity to developing hulled hempseed. As of the writing of this book, just two hulled hempseed products have hit the market: HempNut, from HempNut Incorporated and Nutiva from Kenex. HempNut is now available retail in nitrogen-sealed 12-ounce resealable cans. The sample that I tried was unique in texture and takes on seasonings well. Although small bits of hull can be detected, the meat had an overall softness with only a trace of grit.

My initial concern about hulled hempseed was running the risk of free-radical oxidation. After all, the hull that protects the delicate germ has been removed, exposing it to the elements that destroy its oils. However, as long as the fresh seed is processed at a low temperature and packaged immediately in an oxygen-free container, the product should have a shelf life of over a year.

After exposing hulled hempseed to oxygen, be sure to exercise the same care you do with hempseed oil. It will store well in a sealed container in the refrigerator or freezer for a few weeks. When it does go rancid, there will be a noticeable odor, foul taste, and discoloration. The color of fresh hulled hempseed is bright off-white. When it goes bad, it yellows, then browns.

HempNut is certified organic by the Demeter Organization of Europe and has not been sterilized or fumigated. Obviously, dehulling will prevent the seed from germinating, thereby satisfying U.S. regulations. Since the traces of THC that have shown up in urine tests (see "Free To Pee THC" on page 146) reside on the hull, no traces have been detected in HempNut. This eliminates the risk of testing positive from ingestion of it. HempNut, Inc. guarantees the product to be free of THC.

Because the hull is removed from the equation, the percentages of essential nutrients are higher. The protein content goes up 8 percent (to more than 30 percent) and the total fat content goes up 17 percent (to more than 47 percent). The ratio of essential fatty acids (LA:LNA) remains 3:1. Oddly enough, the content of carbohydrates goes down drastically, from 35 percent to around 10 percent. This may indicate significant carbohydrate content in the hull. Lab analyses should be conducted on the hull itself to verify this. For nutritional analyses, see page 17.

Not only is hempseed one of the most nutrionally complete foods, with the hull removed it is also one of the most versatile. These are just a few of the possible tasty applications: oil, butter, ice cream, chocolate, cheese, burgers, baked goods, confections, prepared meals, pasta, spreads, pâté, chips, dips, beverages, cereal, candy bars, protein drinks, dressings, shakes, and smoothies.

HEMPSEED BUTTER

The vision that drove me to start Hungry Bear Hemp Foods was the production of hempseed butter. I dove right into researching and experimenting with various grinding techniques. I found one machine after another inadequate to the task.

I finally came up with a good process—which required up to $75,000 in equipment. That's when I made the switchover from R&D to production of Seedy Sweeties (hempseed candy bars) to generate revenue to start up my hempseed butter project.

In the autumn of 1996 I worked out a similar process with a local food producer and began production. One process involved grinding whole seed, while the other involved taking nonsterilized pressed hempseed, reconstituting it with oil, and using a special process to grind it into a fine butter. This allowed for the use of any edible oil to create a variety of unique-tasting hempseed butters.

The result was a butter with a rich nutty taste and a consistency and texture much like tahini. Because I was using the whole seed, the pigment from the hull gave it a deep, dark green color.

Now that hulled hempseed is available, it is the obvious ingredient for making hempseed butter. The color is much lighter (due to lack of the pigment-rich hull), the texture is creamier, the protein and essential fatty acid content is higher, the taste is improved, and producing it requires only basic kitchen equipment.

Hulled hempseed butter is so simple to make that you can make it at home with a Champion juicer. Remove the screen, install the blank, and place a bowl under the hub. Run the hulled hempseed through the machine three to five times. The more times you run it through, the more liquefied it will become. Be sure to clean the shaft when you are done—there is over a quarter cup of valuable hempseed butter packed in there.

If you don't have a Champion juicer, there are other options, but it may come out much drier. Make three to four cups at a time in a food processor. A hand-cranked food grinder with a small-holed or flour plate works well. The hempseed kernel is so soft that anything you have that grinds may work.

There are many devices available to small food producers and restaurants that will make quality hempseed butter. For example, a Hobart vertical chopper-mixer or food grinder attachment for the mixer does a splendid job. The butter may need to be run through a few times to achieve the desired consistency. Grinders that rotate at higher speeds tend to liberate more oil, producing a more fluid butter.

As you would expect, it is important to keep hempseed butter sealed and refrigerated when not in use.

You can use hempseed butter as you would tahini. It is a great ingredient in sauces and spreads, works well in shakes and smoothies, is decadent in desserts, and goes well with dried fruit like dates and figs.

The only hempseed butter on the market as of this printing is Hempini, produced by Deer Garden Foods in Santa Cruz, California (see appendix 1). Made from nonsterilized hulled hempseed, it is ground at low temperature, that is, below 119°F(48°C), and packaged in dated glass jars. You can order directly, but better yet, get your local natural food store or co-op to carry it and make this revolutionary product available to your community!

SPROUTED HEMPSEED

Another way to dehull hempseed is to sprout it! Just feed it water and the hulls will pop off by themselves. Sprouting is also a great way to improve nutritional value, transform texture and taste, and increase food mass.

The whole nutritional picture of the seed changes when you sprout it. Since the germ consumes the albumin protein for its initial jump-start of energy, there's less protein for you. However, the sprout does contain active, living enzymes. When photosynthesis begins, green nutrients will be synthesized and available for your nourishment. I look forward to verifying the differences in nutritional value between sprouted and nonsprouted hempseed with comparative analyses.

Sprouting is easy to do at home, provided you live in a country where viable hempseed is legal and available. In a quart jar with a screen-mesh lid, soak 2 heaping tablespoons of viable hempseed overnight. Strain out the water and leave the jar upside down, allowing excess water to drip out. Rinse and strain two or three times a day. The seed should begin germinating within two days. When you see the first green leaves appear, the seed is ready to be eaten. By then the hulls should have separated from the sprouts. If your mesh screen is the right size, the hulls will shake out while you rinse. The water that you strained out contains some nutrients, so recycle it by watering your houseplants with it.

Sprouts can be used fresh in salads and sandwiches. You can also dehydrate them and grind into flour.

PART 2

Hempseed in a Garden of Healing Foods

There is a magic when we both garden and cook. The thoughts, intentions, and energies that we give to our food in garden and kitchen transform and amplify within us when ingested. The songs we sang when we double-dug the beds resound when we crunch into the carrots grown there.

Although hempseed is a complete and splendiferous food, we must be sure to include other foods in our diet. Fortunately, Gaia has bestowed upon us thousands of other edible plants. After years of amalgamating hempseed with every food I've encountered, I have come to the realization that in the appropriate form (oil, butter, flour), hempseed is a universal food complement!

I have chosen to omit the following terms from each ingredient listed in each recipe: "organically grown," "wild harvested," "as local, fresh, natural, and lovingly farmed as possible." I am assuming that you have already made it a priority to nourish yourself with foods of such quality. If you need to learn more about the important role our diets play in the health of our bodies and our planet, check out the suggested reading in appendix 2.

Also remember that if a recipe calls for you to add the "remaining ingredients," then do so in the order listed.

Now, let's take a walk through Earth's gardens to see how each group of fruits, veggies, and fungi can be used with hempseed.

Symbols Used with Recipes

Hempseed oil

Hempseed flour

Hempseed butter

Whole hempseed

Hulled hempseed

Hempseed cake

Herbs and Spices

Seasoning with Hempseed

BEFORE WE BEGIN OUR WALK I'd like to include some seasoning suggestions that you can use to liven up anything you cook. Herbs and spices add flavor, aroma, and medicinal benefits to our food. They should be used as subtle additions though, never dominating or covering up the flavor of the main ingredient.

Since nearly all recipes in this book channel the magic of herbs and spices in one way or another, I won't note all of them here. What follows are some great ways to use hempseed to enhance as well as carry the flavor and other properties of your seasonings.

Seasoning Blends

I recommend these seasoning blends for the three recipes that follow: Seasoned Roasted Hempseed, Roasted Hempseed Meal Seasoning, and Seasoned Hempseed Oil. These are just a few blends that I've come up with; hopefully you will feel inspired to create your own!

Indian Curry Hot or Mild
Mix turmeric, cumin, coriander, cardamom, and fenugreek, plus a few pinches of cayenne or 1 whole fresh cayenne pepper (hot only).

Chinese
Mix cinnamon, coriander, star anise, ginger, nutmeg, cumin, and clove.

Garden Blend
Mix fresh or dried tarragon, thyme, rosemary, sage, and summer savory.

Another Garden Blend
Mix fresh or dried dill, oregano, lemon balm, marjoram, caraway, and bay leaf.

Mexican—Hot, Mild, or Medium
Mix 1 habañero or jalapeño pepper (hot only), the juice and minced flesh of a small tomato, fresh or dried cilantro, and 1 fresh chili pepper or 1 teaspoon chili powder (medium and hot only).

Tamari-Yeast
Mix tamari, nutritional yeast, and fresh minced or powdered garlic.

Italian
Mix fresh or dried basil, oregano, sage, and garlic.

Garlic-Onion
Mix powdered garlic and onion and a pinch of sea salt.

Seasoned Roasted Hempseed

Although bare roasted hempseed packs a flavor that can stand alone, the addition of spices and seasonings puts a thrill in this simple snack food.

Powdered spices and dried herb seasonings work well for roasted hempseed because they adhere well to the oil that has emerged on the surface of the hull. Excessive dry heat can easily burn or destroy the taste of dried seasonings, so it is best to stir them in immediately after you remove the seed from heat, or in the final seconds of roasting.

The power, aroma, and taste of herbs and spices are strongest when freshly ground. It's a good habit to acquire whole dried herbs and spices and grind them on demand with tools such as a mortar and pestle or a hand-cranked flour mill.

Try using some fresh or wet seasonings like minced garlic, toasted sesame oil, and bouillon. Water-based seasonings such as tamari are excellent because the water evaporates, leaving the concentrated flavor in among the seed. Make as much as you want!

You can measure up to 3 tablespoons of wet seasonings per cup of roasted hempseed (use only 1 teaspoon per cup if the seasoning is oil-based).

From any of the Seasoning Blends (or one of your own), you can use up to 1 teaspoon of dried herbs per cup of hempseed, or up to 1 heaping tablespoon of moist herbs.

In a wok or skillet over medium heat, combine the wet seasonings with hot freshly roasted hempseed. Reduce the heat to low so that you don't burn or over-cook anything. Stir constantly until the water has evaporated. If you wish to add dried and powdered seasonings, do so just before the last sign of moisture disappears, or mix with the wet seasonings before you add these to the seed.

It's best to eat roasted hempseed fresh off the griddle (when cool enough for your mouth, of course). Otherwise they'll stay fresh for about a week. Refrigeration will dull the flavor.

Roasted Hempseed Meal Seasoning

As I explained in "Hemp Food-Crafting 101," because of its rich flavor and aroma hempseed meal by itself is considered a seasoning. As with most spices and seasonings its unique flavors and actions combine with others to make astonishing mixes. Make as much as you want!

For both of the following methods, refer to the blends in Seasoning Blends on page 50. Use only those mixes with all-dry ingredients. Use a 1:1 ratio of hempseed to the sum of other seasonings, or adjust to your taste.

Method 1: Roast hempseed as described in "Hemp Food-Crafting 101." Coarsely grind the roasted seed in a hand-cranked flour mill, food grinder, or food processor. Grind other seasonings separately in a mortar and pestle or a mill. Mix together.

Method 2: Combine whole seasonings with hempseed and grind them all together using any tool mentioned in method 1. Whole seeds and other "roastable" herbs can be roasted with the hempseed.

These mixes are at their peak of freshness within an hour of roasting and grinding and will stay good for up to a couple of days.

Seasoned Hempseed Oil

You can use any of the dried-herb blends in Seasoning Blends, or invent your own. Start with whole dried herbs whenever possible. Refrain from using herbs that have water content; this will promote the growth of bacteria. With whatever method you like, reduce the herbs to hempseed sized or smaller. For whole seeds, it is best to crack them open or coarsely grind them with a mortar and pestle. Make as much as you want!

In a stainless-steel, ceramic, or glass saucepan, heat any quantity of hempseed oil to 145°F (63°C). Add 2 heaping tablespoons of herbs per cup of oil. Maintain the temperature for 20 minutes by moving the pan off and on the heat. Stir occasionally. This is about the maximum temperature and duration that I feel comfortable about allowing hempseed oil to endure.

Pour the mixture into a sealable glass jar and let it sit for 2 hours. Replace into a clean saucepan and return to 145°F (63°C). Carefully pour the mixture through a stainless-steel strainer into a clean glass jar (opaque, if possible). Squeeze as much oil as possible out of the herbs. Use immediately or seal with an airtight lid, let cool, then refrigerate or freeze. This should last for up to a month if kept cold, out of the light, and sealed tight.

Many recipes in this book either call for one of the Seasoning Blends, or suggest seasoning hempseed oil with one as described in this recipe. Once you get the knack of this process and the blending of herbs, you'll discover countless uses for them.

Garlic in Hempseed Oil

*You can keep this simple preparation in the fridge to pull out as
needed for a flavorful addition to sauces, spreads, and toast.*

*The quality of the garlic you use is important. Be sure to use
well-cured garlic. Fresh and sprouting garlic is too "live" to store
and will spoil rapidly. If you see bubbles or pressure buildup in the
jar, the mix is no longer healthful to eat. Make as much as you
want!*

Garlic cloves, chopped or minced
Hempseed oil
Extra-virgin olive oil

This mixture will last a month in the refrigerator, so peel whatever quantity of
garlic you can easily eat and share in that time.

Chop or mince the garlic cloves. The finer the garlic is cut, the stronger its
flavor will be. Place as much garlic as you can fit into a jar and fill the rest with a
2:1 ratio of hempseed oil to olive oil. Close the lid and place in the fridge overnight
before using. If the oil settles, then top off the jar with more.

Variation: You can also substitute other oils for the olive oil. Try toasted
sesame oil, peanut oil, flax oil, and so on.

Hemp *Mirepoix*

A mirepoix *is a seasoning of cooked, chopped root vegetables and herbs that is used in stews, in stuffings, or as a garnish. Serves 4.*

    3 tablespoons olive oil
    2 carrots, diced
    1 turnip, diced
    1 onion, chopped
    $^1/_2$ teaspoon dried tarragon
    $^1/_4$ teaspoon celery seeds
    $^1/_4$ teaspoon sea salt
    $^1/_4$ teaspoon freshly ground black pepper
    3 tablespoons hempseed oil

Heat the olive oil in a large iron skillet over medium heat. Sauté the veggies over medium heat, stirring occasionally, for 10 minutes. Turn off the heat and stir in the seasonings and hempseed oil.

Friendly Fungus

OUR WALK THROUGH GAIA'S GARDEN will begin in the forests during the season of rest and reemergence, as we northwesterners call it, the middle of the rainy season. The season that lasts nine months. This temperate rain forest climate provides highly attractive conditions for the tastiest of our fleshy little friends, the fungus among us, the 'shroom in tune, the fun-guy, yes—the marvelous mushrooms!

Of course, every bioregion on this planet is blessed with its own unique variety. These living beings shall be praised as high as cannabis for their earth-healing qualities. In their own quiet way, in their own special moist places they do the work that, in one way or another, helps all other life to thrive.

For example, mycorrhizal fungi, such as the scrumptious matsutakes, chanterelles, and truffles, live symbiotically with the roots of various host plants and trees. The mycelium (the organism that produces the mushroom fruiting body) helps by drawing in and concentrating nutrients from afar for the host plant's roots to absorb.[1]

Most of the gourmet species are saprophytes. This class of fungus decomposes dead plant matter, producing nutritious organic matter and returning carbon, hydrogen, nitrogen, and minerals back into the ecosystem for use by all living things.[2] Some common saprophyte species include shiitake, oyster, and white button mushrooms.

There doesn't seem to be much information out there about the nutritional content unique to each wild mushroom. Generally, mushrooms are 90 percent water; their dry weight is mostly protein and carbohydrates. They have very little fat or calories, but they provide B, C, and D vitamins. Our bodies actually use more calories to digest mushrooms than they provide.[3]

Mushrooms are best prepared when freshly picked. However, when the bounty of your foray is bigger than your family's appetite, you can preserve them by dehydrating, canning, pickling, or freezing.

The simplest method of preparing them is by sautéing in your best extra-virgin olive oil. After a few minutes the mushrooms will expel some water. If the moisture puddles to over one-eighth inch deep, strain out the water (save it for soup stock) and continue sautéing. Add a little more oil, then some seasonings like chives, tarragon, green onions, garlic, or a splash of wine. Different varieties will give you different signs that they are done.

Because mushrooms are rich in protein and carbohydrates and are nearly void of fats, hempseed oil is a natural choice for a balanced friendly fungus recipe.

In addition to the mushroom recipes offered here, see Acorn Squash–Chanterelle Delight (page 91) and Winter Squash–Shiitake Soup (page 92).

Tempura Morels

Morels are spring-fruiting (fall-fruiting in the Midwest and North-east) saprophytes that grow in conifer and hardwood forests throughout North America. Their wrinkly ribs and pits provide an enormous surface area for the flavorful tempura batter to cover. Makes enough batter for 10 to 15 mushrooms.

$1/3$ cup whole wheat flour

$1/3$ cup hempseed flour

$1/3$ cup cornmeal

$1/2$ teaspoon paprika

$1/2$ teaspoon ground coriander

$1/2$ teaspoon ground cumin

$1/4$ teaspoon sea salt

$1/2$ cup water

$1/2$ cup Hempen Ale

1 tablespoon kudzu, dissolved in $1/2$ cup water

Sesame oil (use the nontoasted kind)

Fresh or reconstituted morels

A variety of fresh veggies, cut bite-sized; try broccoli, cauliflower, brussels
  sprouts, tofu, carrots, squash, and onions.

Mix the dry ingredients, then stir in water and ale slowly. Add the kudzu solution. If the mixture seems runny to you, then add a tiny bit more wheat flour. If it is too thick to pour, then add a bit of water. Let the batter meditate alone in a cool place for about an hour.

Pour sesame oil up to an inch deep in an iron skillet of suitable size. Heat the oil until a drop of batter sizzles and floats immediately after you drop it in, but not until it's hot enough to smoke. Dip each morel and veggie piece in the batter, covering it entirely. Allow the batter to penetrate the gills of the morels. Gently drop them into the hot oil, filling the skillet without crowding. Turn over for even frying. They are done when they reach a beautiful golden color. Scoop them out with a slotted spoon, or a strainer, and place them in a colander to drip excess oil before serving.

Porta-Rella Burger

Serves 4.

Marinade:
$^1/_4$ cup olive oil
$^1/_4$ cup red wine
$^1/_4$ cup water
1 tablespoon maple syrup
1 tablespoon tamari or Braggs Liquid Aminos
$^1/_4$ teaspoon ground cumin
1 pinch ground black pepper

Burgers:
4 porta bella mushrooms (4–5 inches in diameter)
2 fancy sweet peppers (your choice)
1 4-oz. package of Hemp Rella cheese alternative, grated.
4 whole-wheat burger buns
Lettuce, tomato, sprouts, and other burger fixings.

Combine the marinade ingredients in bowl. Remove the stems from the mushroom caps. Slice the stems thick and leave the caps whole. Remove seeds and stems from peppers and slice into wide wedges. Place mushrooms and peppers into a flat, quart-size sealable container with the mushroom gills facing up. Pour the marinade over them, saturating the gills as much as possible. Let sit for an hour or two.

With the gills facing up, cook the mushrooms and peppers in one or two covered iron skillets on medium-high heat. Add marinade sauce as needed to keep the pan and mushrooms moist. Turn over when mushrooms soften and the side facing the cooking surface browns. When the gill side is done, turn over once more (gills facing up) and cover with grated Hemp Rella. Cover and cook just long enough to melt the Hemp Rella.

Meanwhile toast the buns and dress with burger fixings. Remove mushrooms and peppers from skillet, stack with the fixings on the bun, and serve!

Sesame 'Shroom Dressing

Let the delicious flavors of mushrooms and hempseed add dash to your salads. Makes 1 cup.

1/4 cup rice vinegar
Juice of 1/2 lemon
2 pinches sea salt
2 pinches black pepper, ground
1/2 cup hempseed oil
2 heaping tablespoons tahini
1 tablespoon hempseed butter
1/2 teaspoon reishi mushroom powder*
1/2 teaspoon shiitake mushroom powder*
1/4 teaspoon spirulina powder
1/2 teaspoon cumin powder

Mix all the ingredients together, making sure the hempseed butter and tahini dissolve well. Serve with an equally unique salad.

*Available through health food stores or Asian food markets.

Hempseed Underground:

The Root Vegetables

WHEN I DOUBLE-DIG MY GARDEN BEDS for planting, I like to plunge my hands as far down into that soft, loamy soil as I can and resonate with the root energies.

I feel the moisture and draw nutrients through my fingers up my arms into my soul. I feel a worm tickle my palm. I have many friends down here to keep me company, many microcreatures—we help each other out. I can stay planted here all winter with all my vitality intact. If I'm a bulb or perennial my aerials come back to life when the soil warms up.

I am the root. I serve the earth and her children by caretaking the soil and providing durable nourishment. I am frugal with the energy I store. I grow to contribute to the survival of Earth's children above and below.

Root vegetables and herbs have helped sustain our species for our entire existence. They store well, are easy to grow, and provide a powerhouse of nutrients in the form of complex carbohydrates, fiber, protein, vitamins, and minerals.

Significant quantities of vitamin C can be found in many roots, including sweet potatoes, turnips, and parsnips. Since vitamin C is destroyed by high heat, it is best to eat these veggies raw for maximum retention of this precious nutrient.

Cruciferous roots (those belonging to the mustard family, Cruciferae or Brassicaceae) are known to help ward off cancer.[1] This family includes radishes, horseradish, rutabagas, and turnips.

The more vibrantly orange a root is, the more beta-carotene it contains. Named for the carrot, beta-carotene helps prevent heart disease and is likely to help in the prevention and treatment of cancer. Beta-carotene is a precursor to vitamin A in our bodies. That means it's stored and metabolized into usable vitamin A as our body needs it.

Symptoms of vitamin A deficiency are very similar to those of EFA deficiency. They include split, peeled, and rigid fingernails; dry, brittle, and dull hair; and blemished, wrinkly, and dry skin.

When selecting root veggies, choose roots that are firm and vibrant in color. Avoid those that are soft, dull colored, wrinkled, blemished, hairy, or—in the case of potatoes—have sprouting eyes.

If you garden in cold climates, many roots, such as parsnips, salsify, and horseradish, can spend the winter in the frozen ground. By spring thaw their starch has turned to sugar, giving them a subtly sweet flavor.

When cooking roots with hempseed, it is good to let the dish remain a complex carbohydrate powerhouse by going light on the protein-rich hempseed flour and butter. Roots prefer to be bathed in the oil of hempseed. This oil is the spot of yin in the heart of the yang of root vegetables.

Baked Beets with
Yogurt and Hempseed Oil

Serves 3.

- 3 large beets
- 1 cup soy yogurt
- 2 tablespoons hempseed oil
- $1/4$ cup chives, chopped
- 2 tablespoons dill weed, dried or minced fresh
- 3 pinches sea salt

Preheat the oven to 425°F (218°C). Place the beets, washed but untrimmed, in a covered baking pan and bake for 1 hour. Let the beets cool for a few minutes. Combine the yogurt, hempseed oil, chives, and dill weed in a small bowl. Uncover the beets. With a paring knife, remove their skins and trim them. Mash the beets, sprinkle sea salt over them, and place in three small serving bowls. Plop some of the yogurt—hempseed oil mixture on top of each bowl and serve.

Glazed Shallots with Minced Garlic and Hempseed Oil

Serves 4-6.

20 shallots, peeled
3 tablespoons olive oil
3 tablespoons turbinado sugar
Juice of 1 lemon
$^1/_4$ cup white cooking wine
$^1/_2$ cup Garlic in Hempseed Oil (see recipe on page 54)

Preheat the oven to 350°F (177°C). Place the shallots in a shallow baking dish and brush them with half of the olive oil. Combine 2 tablespoons of the turbinado sugar with the lemon juice and wine in a small bowl. Pour slowly over the shallots then stir them up, coating them well. Bake uncovered for 1 hour. Combine the remaining olive oil and turbinado sugar; splash it over shallots. Continue baking (about half an hour longer) until the liquid has evaporated and the shallots are soft and glossy. Spread the Garlic in Hempseed Oil over the top. Serve as a side dish with a pasta or tofu main course.

Live Root Meal

Serves 4.

  1 carrot, grated
  $^1/_2$ cup beet, grated
  1 six-inch daikon radish, grated
  2 scallion stalks, minced
  $^1/_4$ cup hempseed oil
  2 tablespoons yellow miso
  4 pickle wedges, diced

Combine all ingredients and serve as a side dish, a sandwich filling, or to liven up a salad.

Root Pancakes

These cakes can be served with syrup for breakfast; as veggie-burger patties; or as a side dish with dinner. Serves 6–8.

2 carrots, grated
1 turnip, grated
1 sweet potato, grated
2 white onions, grated
2 heaping tablespoons kudzu root starch dissolved in 1$^{1}/_{2}$ cups water
$^{1}/_{4}$ cup arrowroot powder
1 cup hempseed flour
4 cloves garlic, peeled and minced
1 thumb-sized piece of fresh ginger, grated
$^{1}/_{2}$ teaspoon sea salt
$^{1}/_{4}$ teaspoon freshly ground white pepper
Safflower oil

Combine the grated root veggies in a large mixing bowl. Stir in the remaining ingredients (except the safflower oil). Stir until consistently mixed. Cover and refrigerate for a couple of hours. Oil an iron skillet and heat over a medium-high flame. Stir the batter again. With a ladle, drop the batter onto the skillet, making cakes about 3 inches in diameter. Make sure that the skillet is fully heated, or the cakes may stick. Cook on both sides, flipping when the downside turns golden-brown. Add oil as needed. When both sides are cooked, remove the cake to a covered platter and keep warm in a 250°F (120°C) oven—or serve right off the griddle.

POTATOES

On winter mornings a warm, hefty bowl of hempy spuds will ground you out and power you up with complex carbos. If they're cooked thoroughly, that is—for undercooked potatoes are so difficult for the body to break down that simply digesting them may hog all the energy you would prefer using for your day's activities. Like lots of work, but no pay. It's best not to allow underdone potatoes past your lips. If you eat out, make sure your spuds are done: when restaurants get busy, they often decrease the cooking time of their potatoes. The resulting heavy-bellied, sluggish customer ends up washing the meal down with coffee to force the adrenals to compensate for the missing food energy.

I might as well take this opportunity to warn you about green potatoes. They contain a toxin called solanine, which may cause illness. Exposure to sunlight causes potatoes to turn green and produce solanine. So just say no to green potatoes.

Since a potato-based dish will be very starchy and high in carbohydrates, keep any protein additions (hempseed flour or butter) to a minimum; instead, use oil as the main hemp component. If taters are cut up and baked, deep-fried, or skillet-fried, cook until edges begin to brown.

Spuds Done Hempy

The persecution of plants and foods is no new thing. Soon after South American potatoes took root in Europe a fifteenth-century pope denounced them as an erotic stimulant. During the Renaissance potatoes were publicly burned to protect the population from the plant that supposedly carried leprosy, rickets, and warts.

Sound like reefer madness? *Or in this case,* tuber lunacy. *Seems the control freaks of each era choose a different plant to diabolize. Serves 3.*

$^1/_2$ garlic bulb, peeled and diced
1 medium yellow onion, diced
1 green bell pepper, chopped
4 large potatoes, cut into bite-sized chunks
Safflower oil
$^1/_4$ cup hempseed flour
2 pinches sea salt
2 pinches black pepper
$^1/_4$ teaspoon paprika
$^1/_4$ teaspoon celery seed
$^1/_4$ cup hempseed oil
2 tablespoons tamari
$^1/_4$ cup nutritional yeast

In an oiled skillet over a medium-high flame, sauté the onions, garlic, and bell pepper until browned. Meanwhile, place the cut-up potatoes in a separate oiled skillet over a medium-high flame and cover. After a minute, stir the potatoes, stirring in a bit more safflower oil. Reduce the heat to medium, cover, and continue stirring the potatoes every minute or so. When they begin to soften up after about 15 minutes, add the hempseed flour and seasonings, stirring these well into the potatoes. When the potato edges start to brown, they are beginning to be done. Cook them longer if you like them well done. Stir in hempseed oil, tamari, and yeast—along with everything from the other skillet—and serve.

Mashed Sweet Potatoes

Sweet potatoes (Ipomoea batatas) *are not potatoes, but a tuber in the morning-glory (Convolvulaceae) family. Although they're often called yams, the two plants are unrelated. Sweet potatoes are native to Central America; yams are native to Africa and make up the genus* Dioscorea *of the family Dioscoreaceae. Sweet potatoes are nutritionally superior to yams and blend very well with hempseed oil. Serves 4.*

4 large sweet potatoes
Olive oil
1 teaspoon ground Jamaican allspice
2 pinches sea salt
$^1/_2$ cup coconut milk
$^1/_4$ cup hempseed oil

Preheat the oven to 425°F (218°C). Wash, scrub, and dry the sweet potatoes, then rub all over with olive oil. Pop them into the oven on a cookie sheet, uncovered. Bake about 45 minutes, until inserting a knife shows that they're soft all the way through. Place them in a sturdy mixing bowl and mash, removing large pieces of skin if they are bothersome. Mash in the remaining ingredients. Serve as a side dish; try topping with a yogurt sauce.

Legumes

LEGUMES ARE A FAMILY OF PLANTS whose fruits are seed-carrying pods. Included in the legume family are peas, peanuts, beans of all sorts, clover, Scots broom, and alfalfa.

The edible legumes nourish our bodies by supplying us with a wealth of protein. They are good survival food, too, because they store easily for a long time.

They serve the soil well by helping fix nitrogen into it. Actually, symbiotic bacteria called rhizobium do the nitrogen fixation. These bacteria form nodules on the roots and convert molecular atmospheric nitrogen (the most abundant gas in our air) to a compound that is absorbable by the roots of plants. Nitrogen is one of the three primary nutrients needed for plant growth (nitrogen, phosphorus, and potassium). It is important for plants' early stages of rapid growth and can be depleted from the soil if not replenished (by nitrogen-fixing plants, manure, or soil amendments).

For these reasons, growing legumes in rotation with other crops is a boon for both the health of the soil and the balance of our diets. Cover crops (cutting or tilling plants into the soil before they mature) or food crops (harvested seeds) of legumes will leave the soil rich in nitrogen and full of organic matter (if the rest of the plant goes back to the soil). Common legume cover crops include fava beans, vetch, cowpeas (black-eyed peas), soybeans, and many varieties of clover.

One year I planted carrots under the snow peas to see if they would be good companion plants. The carrots were fed so well by the nitrogen from the peas that they quickly took over the whole pea patch.

Rotating legumes with other food crops also works well to balance our food supply and our nutritional needs. If your soil is producing legumes two seasons of the year and fresh food the other two, your harvest may very well be in balance with your rate and ratio of consumption.

Because they're high in protein, hempseed flour and butter make delicious companions to legumes. I've never gone wrong adding hempseed oil to any bean dish either. Not only do their tastes and textures complement each other nicely, but consuming them together enhances the body's metabolism as well.

The basic method for cooking beans is to first soak them in a generous amount of water overnight, then strain. (The soaking water is rich in nitrogen, so save it for your plants.) In a pot, bring beans and fresh water to a boil. For every cup of dry beans, use four cups of water. Reduce heat and simmer for four hours. Lentils and split peas do not need to soak and take less than an hour to cook.

Hemp-Lentil Loaf

Lentils are versatile, are easy to sprout (they germinate in a day and have outstanding taste, texture, and nutrition), and take as little as a half hour to cook. Just see what happens to the flavor and texture of cooked lentils when you add lots of hempseed flour and oil! Garlic, onions, salt, miso, and Indian spices liven up the hearty and grounded lentil-hempseed combination. To prevent blackening and taste deterioration, I leave lentils out of iron pots.

I like to serve this loaf to meat eaters to show them how vegan grub can stick to the ribs! Serves 6–10.

9 cups water, with a pinch of sea salt
3 cups dry lentils
1 cup hempseed flour
1 heaping tablespoon kelp powder
1 heaping tablespoon onion powder
1 teaspoon paprika
1 teaspoon baking powder
1/4 teaspoon sea salt
1/4 cup corn oil
1/2 garlic bulb, peeled and diced
1 fresh chili pepper, diced very fine (or 1 teaspoon chili powder)
Plain or seasoned hempseed oil of your choice.

Preheat the oven to 375°F (190°C). In a large stainless-steel pot, bring the water to a boil. Add the lentils and return to a boil. Lower heat and simmer for 45 minutes.

Strain excess water, if any, by pouring the whole mixture into a colander over a large bowl. Save liquid for future soup stock, and return the lentils to the pot (with the burner off). Stir in the remaining ingredients (except the hempseed oil). Spoon into two well-oiled loaf pans and bake for 45 minutes. Top with your choice of plain or seasoned hempseed oil (see page 53) and serve with a saucy dish.

Muddy River Marinated Tofu with Green Island Sauce

Serves 3.

- 1 pound firm tofu, cut into bite-sized chunks (be creative!)
- 3 tablespoons balsamic vinegar
- 3 tablespoons tamari
- 2 tablespoons Dr. Bronner's Mineral Bouillon
- 1 tablespoon hempseed oil
- 2 heaping tablespoons hempseed flour
- 1 heaping tablespoon kelp powder
- 2 tablespoons American ginseng extract
- 2 cups Green Island Sauce (see recipe on page 95; I prefer it cold for this recipe)

Place the tofu chunks in a resealable quart container with a wide mouth. Pour the vinegar into a small bowl then stir in, one at a time, the remaining ingredients, except Green Island Sauce. Pour this mixture over the tofu and seal the container. Gently give it a tumbling gravity swirl until the tofu is well coated. Set the container aside, on its side, tumbling it occasionally. It is best to prepare this a few hours before serving and leave at room temperature to let it fully marinate.

Serve over a bed of steamed basmati rice and grated carrot, lightly seasoned with yellow mustard seeds. Spoon the marinated tofu on one side and the Green Island Sauce on the other.

Spicy Hemp-Bean Dip

You can use this as a dip for veggies, chips, rice cakes, or bread—or as sandwich spread or burrito filling. Makes 4 cups.

    1 cup dry beans (any combination of pinto, black, lentil, mung, or
        adzuki beans)
    4 cups water
    $^1/_2$ teaspoon sea salt
    $^1/_4$ teaspoon paprika
    $^1/_4$ teaspoon celery seeds
    $^1/_4$ teaspoon brown mustard powder
    $^1/_4$ teaspoon ground allspice
    5 garlic cloves, peeled and minced
    1 or 2 fresh red chili peppers (or substitute $^1/_4$ to $^1/_2$ teaspoon chili
        powder)
    $^1/_2$ bell pepper, diced
    $^1/_4$ cup hempseed flour
    $^1/_4$ cup hempseed oil

Soak the beans in the water for 4 hours in a pot. Bring to a boil, then reduce the heat and simmer for 2 hours. Strain out all excess liquid by pouring the beans into a colander over a bowl. Save bean juice for future soup stock. Place the beans and the remaining ingredients in a food processor. Blend on high for 3 minutes. Chill before serving.

Hemp-Garbanzo Spread

This spread is delicious on whole wheat pita bread. Makes 6–8 cups, depending on size of summer squash.

3 cups garbanzo beans, cooked or sprouted
$^1/_2$ cup hempseed butter
$^1/_2$ cup tahini
$^1/_4$ cup hempseed oil
Juice of 1 lemon
1 jalapeño pepper, diced
4 garlic cloves, peeled and diced
$^1/_4$ teaspoon ground cayenne
$^1/_4$ teaspoon ground cumin
2 pinches sea salt
$^1/_2$ cup green onions, chopped
1 medium carrot, grated
2 medium yellow summer squash, grated

In a large, sturdy bowl, mash the beans. Continue to mash in the remainder of the ingredients. Serve in a decorative bowl garnished with a couple of sprigs of parsley. This recipe also works well with a food processor if you have one.

Split Pea Spread

Spread this great dip on sandwiches, crackers, and veggies.
Makes 1 cup.

    1 cup cooked split peas (refrigerated or leftover split pea soup)
    $1/4$ cup hempseed oil
    2 small garlic cloves, peeled and minced
    1 teaspon yellow mustard powder
    $1/4$ teaspoon paprika
    $1/2$ teaspoon kelp powder

Combine all ingredients, stir well, and serve!

From the Sea

I HAVE DREAMED FOR A LONG TIME of running a vegan seafood restaurant. The slogan would be a variation of an old cliché: "There's more than just fish in the ocean."

Given the severe mineral depletion that has taken place in cropland soil, we must go to the sea for mineral-rich sea veggies.

Unless you are fortunate enough to acquire them freshly harvested, the sea veggies you find in the store will most likely be dehydrated. After a quick rinse, you can help them regain their tender texture by soaking them in water, tamari, or a flavorful marinade. Powdered or flaked sea veggies can be used as a dry seasoning in a moist dish.

Dulse Delight

Supreme 7 is a marvelous blend of seven nutritious oils: hemp, flax, sesame, poppy, pumpkin, pomegranate, and sunflower. It was created by Herbal Products and Development; see appendix 1 for more information. Makes 1 cup to add to 4 to 6 servings of udon noodles or cooked grains.

2 ounces dulse flakes

Water

Handful of shallots, peeled and minced

$^1/_2$ cup walnuts, chopped

5 tablespoons Supreme 7 (or your own blend of hempseed, flax, and
  other nutritious oils)

2 heaping tablespoons kelp powder

$^1/_2$ teaspoon celery seeds

Place the dulse in a small bowl and stir in just enough water to consistently moisten it; don't get the mixture soggy. Let this sit for 10 minutes. Stir in the remaining ingredients.

Broiled Land and Sea Tofu

Years of experience cooking deep-sea fish went into the creation of this vegan mock-fish recipe. Serves 2.

Juice of 1 lemon

$^1/_2$ cup water

8 asparagus spears

1 pound tofu, soft

$^1/_2$ medium carrot, grated

$^1/_2$ teaspoon yellow mustard powder

1 tablespoon kelp powder

1 teaspoon chopped fresh sage

1 teaspoon chopped fresh thyme

1 teaspoon chopped fresh rosemary

1 pound cauliflower, cut into bite-sized pieces

$^1/_4$ pound oyster mushrooms (you can substitute any mushrooms if oysters are unavailable)

$^1/_2$ to $^1/_4$ teaspoon fenugreek

$^1/_2$ to $^1/_4$ teaspoon ground turmeric

$^1/_2$ to $^1/_4$ teaspoon paprika

$^1/_2$ teaspoon ground cumin

Pinch sea salt

2 teaspoons olive oil

6 tablespoons Seasoned Hempseed Oil (see recipe on page 53) made with any of the Seasoning Blends (see recipes on page 50)

Preheat the broiler. Mix together the lemon juice and water in a 16-ounce cup or jar. Bend the asparagus spears until each one snaps in two. Compost the bottoms, and soak the tops in the jar of lemon water while you prepare the rest of the recipe. Mash together the tofu, carrot, mustard, kelp, sage, thyme, and rosemary. Spread this mixture onto two single-serving size broiling pans. Into the tofu base, stuff in small pieces of cauliflower, then mushrooms; place the asparagus on top. With a mortar and pestle, grind together the spices and sea salt. Sprinkle on top of the tofu and veggies. Slowly pour the lemon water over everything, especially the mushrooms. Place under the broiler for 15 to 20 minutes. Check from time to time and remove from broiler when vegetables are easily pierced by a fork and lightly browned. Pour Seasoned Hempseed Oil over everything and serve!

Hemp Land and Sea Spread

Paul Gaylon from Herbal Products and Development offers this delightful sandwich spread recipe. It's one of many recipes Paul has been compiling for his upcoming book, The Hempseed Uncook Book, *which will highlight the benefits of raw foods and fresh, unheated hemp oil. Makes 5 cups.*

2 tablespoons hempseed oil
Dash of medium-spicy hot sauce
1 heaping tablespoon vegetable powder or Dr. Bronner's Seasoning Mix
Sprinkle of red dulse flakes
2 tablespoons flax oil
1 heaping tablespoon pumpkin seeds, diced
Knifeful of whole-grain mustard
$1^1/_2$ teaspoons Bragg's Liquid Aminos
1 small lemon
1 pound firm tofu
1 small red onion, minced
Sprinkle of ground sesame seeds
$^1/_8$ teaspoon caraway seeds

Just mix it all up and spread it on bagels, breads, or crackers.

Veggies and Grains

AHOY LANDLUBBERS! We've come ashore from that brief cruise seaward with an appetite for the hearty fare that grows on terra firma.

VEGGIE FRUITS

You've probably encountered that trick question, "Is a tomato a fruit or a vegetable?" The trickster may have been hoping you would fall for it by replying, "Vegetable."

Well, the trick is on the trickster because the way I see it, the correct answer is "Both! A tomato is a fruit, and all fruits are vegetables." To take it a step further, you could also prove that a tomato is technically a berry. If you really wanted to show off, you could write the word TOMATO vertically in capital letters. Then hold it to a mirror and see what it says.

A *vegetable*, simply put, is any edible portion of a plant. A *fruit* is a structure produced by a plant that is often fleshy and edible. It houses one or more ripened ovaries and comes in various forms. Not only do tomatoes fit this definition, but so do peppers, squash, cucumbers, eggplants, and legumes. They all go well with our favorite fruit: hempseed!

I like to call these friends Veggie Fruits because by recognizing them as fruits, we empower the fertility of the food.

Jai High Stuffed Peppers

Serves 3.

2 tablespoons toasted sesame oil

2 or more tablespoons safflower oil

2 fingers fresh turmeric, grated (or 1 heaping tablespoon ground)

$^1/_2$ garlic bulb, peeled and minced

$^1/_2$ teaspoon fenugreek

1$^1/_3$ cups quinoa

$^2/_3$ cup millet

$^2/_3$ cup amaranth

5$^1/_3$ cups water

1 carrot, grated

$^1/_3$ cup sesame seeds

$^1/_3$ cup sunflower seeds

1 heaping tablespoon hempseed butter

$^1/_3$ cup brown rice syrup

3 red or yellow bell peppers

Garlic in Hempseed Oil (see recipe on page 54)

In a saucepan over medium-high heat, heat the sesame and safflower oils. Add the turmeric, garlic, and fenugreek. Swirl around. When the fenugreek starts crackling, add the grains. Stir to cover the grains in oil. Reduce the heat to medium, and add the water and carrot. Bring to a boil, lower heat, and steam for 20 minutes.

Preheat the oven to 425°F (218°C). Grind up the sesame and sunflower seeds in a food grinder or processor. In a mixing bowl, combine the ground seeds, 1$^1/_2$ cups of the cooked grain, the hempseed butter, and the brown rice syrup. Stir. Cut off the stem end of each pepper like a jack-o'-lantern and remove the seeds. Stuff each pepper with the mixture. In an oiled iron skillet or bread pan, form a bed of the rest of the cooked grains. Nest the stuffed peppers into the bed of grains. Bake for 30 minutes, then serve with a generous topping of Garlic in Hempseed Oil.

Vegan Hempseed Stuffed Shells

Serves 4-6.

4 cups tomato sauce
1 pound firm tofu
$^1/_4$ cup hempseed oil
$^1/_4$ cup tahini
Juice of $^1/_2$ lemon
2 tablespoons hempseed butter
2 heaping tablespoons minced garlic
2 heaping tablespoons minced pine nuts
$^1/_4$ cup minced scallions
$^1/_2$ cup fresh basil, chopped
Splash of balsamic vinegar
Palmful of oregano
1 teaspoon dill weed, dried or minced fresh
$^1/_2$ cup sliced black olives
8 ounces large pasta shells

Preheat the oven to 350°F (177°F). In a small saucepan, bring the tomato sauce to a simmer and keep warm until ready to use. Meanwhile, mash the tofu in a large bowl. Add the remainder of the ingredients (except the pasta) one at a time while mashing and stirring.

Bring a potful of water to a boil and add the pasta shells. Return to a boil and cook 10 to 15 minutes to taste; strain and rinse with cold water. With a tablespoon, stuff each shell with the tofu mixture and place close together in a lasagna pan. Slowly pour the tomato sauce over the shells, cover with foil, and bake for 35 minutes. Serve warm.

Garden Pasta Salad

Serves 4-6.

    1 medium cucumber
    6 tablespoons hempseed oil
    6 tablespoons tahini
    10 heaping tablespoons soy yogurt
    4 cups fancy ribbon pasta
    3 cups sugar snap peas, stems pinched off

Slice the cucumber in half lengthwise and scoop out the core from both halves. Do not peel unless the cucumber has been waxed. Chop the inner core into bite-sized pieces and set aside. Then dice the outer part of the cuke, reserving separately.

In a small bowl, make a sauce by stirring the hempseed oil and tahini into the soy yogurt, then adding chopped cuke core. Blend well.

Bring a large potful of water to a boil, then add the pasta. Reduce the heat and cook for a few minutes to soften the pasta.

Strain the parboiled pasta, saving the straining water. Replace the pasta into the pot along with 2 cups of the water. Add peas and diced outer cukes. Cook over low heat for 10 minutes. Strain out any remaining cooking water and rinse with cold water. Place in a serving bowl, toss with the sauce, and serve!

Nutty Avocado Salad

Serves 4.

2 medium avocados, diced or mashed, depending on ripeness
Juice of 1 lemon
$^1/_2$ teaspoon dried dillweed
1 tablespoon chives (fresh if possible)
$^1/_2$ teaspoon sage (fresh if possible)
1 pinch cayenne powder
3 medium celery stalks, chopped
1 medium carrot, grated
$^1/_2$ cup chopped cabbage
$^1/_4$ cup diced onion
1 cup cashews, ground
$^1/_4$ cup hempseed oil
6 cups sprouts or other greens

Prepare and mix all ingredients (except the sprouts or greens) in a large bowl. Stir it up and serve on a bed of sprouts or greens.

WINTER SQUASH

Winter squash is an essential crop for those intent on living off their garden all year long. When stored properly (cool and dry), most varieties will last until spring. These veggie fruits are generally powerhouses of complex carbohydrates, potassium, and vitamin A as well, making them great companions to hempseed—especially hempseed oil. Hempseed butter and hempseed oil both beautifully complement the hearty and naturally sweet flavor of most winter squash. You'll find that mushrooms and winter squash are natural companions as well. The next two recipes combine all three flavors—squash, mushrooms, and hempseed—into hearty, flavorful fare perfect for the colder months. See also Winter Squash Pie Filling on page 117.

I've found that baking is the best method of preparation for retaining winter squash's taste, texture, and nutrients. For squash that is generally roundish (such as acorn or hubbard), cut in half through the equator. For those that are more elongated (such as delicata or butternut), cut in half through the longitudinal center. Scoop out the seeds, and bake at 425°F (218°C), facedown on a cookie sheet for 30 to 50 minutes, depending on size.

The skin of most winter squash is too tough to be edible, although that of smaller squash such as delicatas may be tender enough for eating. Test a piece of the squash you are cooking and decide for yourself.

The sweet, hearty, and satisfying taste of winter squash lends itself to simple dishes. It's easy to make a meal out of a squash fresh from the oven—just place it in a bowl and mash up the flesh with a fork. Add a few tablespoons of hempseed oil and a little squirt of Dr. Bronner's Mineral Bouillon. Enjoy!

Don't waste those seeds! In the same way that winter squash extends your food supply through the winter, planting the seeds in the spring extends *its* life. Just rinse the flesh off the seeds as best you can, then soak in water for about a month, stirring every day to prevent foul decay. Finally, rinse off the seeds once more really well, discarding any that have split open or gone to mush. Dry the seeds with very little heat (less than 100°F [38°C]) and lots of airflow until they're completely dry. They can be dried in a food dehydrator, or in the sun. They will dry in 48 hours or so depending on the drying method used. Store in a cool, dry place until spring planting.

If you feel you would rather *eat* the seeds, just rinse them off and roast them in a 425°F (218°C) oven on a cookie sheet until golden. Sprinkle over a dish or eat them straight.

Acorn Squash–
Chanterelle Delight

Serves 2-3.

- 2¹/₄ pounds acorn squash
- 10 tablespoons hempseed oil
- 2 teaspoons ground cumin (or replace the hempseed oil and ground cumin with 10 tablespoons of already prepared cumin-spiced hempseed oil; see recipe on page 50)
- 2 tablespoons bee pollen
- ¹/₄ cup pine nuts
- 1 tablespoon safflower oil
- ¹/₄ pound fresh chanterelle mushrooms, cut into bite-sized pieces

Cut the squash in half (save the seeds for planting), and bake it at 425°F (218°C) for 35 minutes. Meanwhile, pour the hempseed oil into a small saucepan and warm it over medium heat for 1 minute. Remove from the heat and add the cumin and bee pollen. Let the mixture sit, covered.

In an iron skillet, brown the pine nuts over medium-high heat. Add the safflower oil. After 15 seconds, add the chanterelles; keep stirring and turning until they are tender and golden and the water has evaporated. Remove from the heat and pour into the saucepan with the hempseed oil. Stir and cover. When the squash is done, scoop out the meat from the skin into a large bowl. Mash it up with a potato masher, then mold the squash into a bowl shape and fill the center with the mushroom mixture. Serve immediately.

Winter Squash–
Shiitake Soup

Any soup can be hempified simply by adding a tablespoon of hempseed oil to each bowl just before serving. Because heat will accelerate fatty acid degeneration, it would be unwise to cook hempseed oil with the rest of the soup. Serves 6–8.

5 pounds winter squash of your choice, seeded and cut into chunks
1 heaping tablespoon kudzu root starch dissolved in 1 cup water
2 heaping tablespoons minced fresh ginger
$^1/_4$ cup hempseed butter
1 garlic bulb, peeled and minced
1 yellow onion, chopped into chunks
$^1/_4$ cup olive oil
2 cups shiitake mushrooms, cut into bite-sized chunks
1 carrot, grated
1 turnip, grated
1 teaspoon kelp powder
1 teaspoon celery seeds
Hempseed oil
Natto miso

In a large pot, boil 8 cups of water. Add the squash chunks, reduce the heat, cover and simmer, stirring occasionally, for 20 minutes or until soft. If the squash skin is not edible, then remove squash chunks, skin them, and return to pot (be careful—they're hot!). Add 9 cups of water and return to a boil, then reduce the heat to a simmer. Add the dissolved kudzu, ginger, and hempseed butter. In an iron skillet, sauté the garlic and onion in the olive oil. When they begin to brown, throw in the shiitakes and sauté until the onions caramelize, then add to the soup. Add the grated carrot, turnip, kelp powder, and celery seed. Continue stirring and cooking until the squash has fully dissolved and has thickened the soup. Serve with a tablespoon each of hempseed oil and natto miso in each bowl.

GRAINS

The basic way to cook grains is to bring 2 to 3 cups of water to a boil, add 1 cup of dry grain, bring to a boil again, reduce heat to low, cover, and cook until the pot stops steaming. Rice will take 35 to 40 minutes to cook, while quinoa will take as little as 20 to 30 minutes. *The New Laurel's Kitchen* cookbook includes a good table on cooking grains, giving relative proportions of grain to water and cooking times for a wide variety of grains (see appendix 2, "Suggested Reading").

Since grains are usually very high in carbohydrates, balance them by minimizing the use of high-protein forms of hempseed like flour and butter. Instead, it's palatable and sensible to bathe grain dishes in hempseed oil. A simple bowl of cooked grain, such as quinoa, millet, amaranth, or brown rice sprinkled with nutritional yeast and doused with hempseed oil and tamari, makes a satisfying dish. Or you might want to build a meal around a whole grain, fresh veggies, and one of the sauces or dressings offered in the next section.

Swami Seasoned Veggie Rice

Serves 3-4.

3 tablespoons peanut oil
1 teaspoon fenugreek
1 teaspoon ground turmeric
1 teaspoon whole brown mustard seeds
1 teaspoon whole cumin seeds
2 cups basmati rice
1 medium carrot, grated
1 cup shredded green cabbage
1 baseball-sized pattypan squash
4 cups water
4 tablespoons hempseed oil

Pour the peanut oil into a 2-quart pot over medium-high heat. Add the seasonings and swirl until consistently coated. When the seeds begin to pop, reduce the heat to medium and stir in the rice and veggies, coating them with oil. After 1 minute return the heat to medium-high, add the water, cover, and bring to a boil; turn the heat down to low and steam for 35 minutes. Add hempseed oil just before serving.

SAUCES AND DRESSINGS FOR VEGGIES AND GRAINS

The next six recipes provide versatile toppings for any number of grain, pasta, and veggie dishes. See also Sesame 'Shroom Dressing on page 60.

Green Island Sauce

This is a tasty sauce for pasta and grains—as well as for Muddy River Marinated Tofu (see recipe on page 74). Serves 4.

$^1/_4$ pound fresh green beans
1 medium zucchini
1$^1/_2$ cups coconut milk
1 cup fresh cilantro
6 tablespoons hempseed oil

In a metal steaming basket or bamboo or ceramic steamer, cook the beans and zuke for 10 minutes. Meanwhile, warm the coconut milk in a saucepan. In a blender or food processor, puree the green beans, zuke, coconut milk, and cilantro until smooth. Allow to cool in the blender for 30 minutes. Add the hempseed oil. Blend for another 30 seconds and serve.

Coconut-Veggie Sauce
for Cooked Grains

Serves 2-4.

1^1/$_2$ cups coconut milk
Finger-sized chunk of fresh ginger, peeled and chopped
1 heaping tablespoon red curry paste or powder
^{1}/$_4$ pound fresh green beans
Golf-ball-sized chunk of Jerusalem artichoke, quartered
1 medium carrot
2 tablespoons hempseed oil
1 tangerine

In a saucepan, bring the coconut milk to a boil, then reduce the heat to a simmer. Add the ginger and red curry paste. Steam the green beans, Jerusalem artichoke, and carrot for 10 minutes. Swirl the veggies and coconut milk in a blender on high speed. Add the hempseed oil and the juice of half of the tangerine; blend until smooth. Serve over rice, quinoa, or pasta. Slice the rest of the tangerine and serve on the side.

Zesty Spring Dressing for Steamed Veggies

This dressing is great poured over fresh-steamed veggies such as fava beans, green beans, kale, chard, asparagus, or leeks atop a bed of rice or quinoa. Makes $^3/_4$ cup that would cover 4–6 heaping servings of steamed veggies.

$^1/_4$ cup hempseed oil
Juice of 3 lemons
$^1/_4$ cup olive oil
1 teaspoon dried alfalfa leaf
1 teaspoon dried dill
$^1/_4$ teaspoon kelp powder
Pinch sea salt

Combine all ingredients in a bottle or jar. Shake it up and serve!

Winter Salad Sauce

When big chunks of veggies are dressed in a hearty sauce, a salad can become a meal. In the colder months you can warm up a cool salad with this spicy dressing. A split pea or mung bean soup would complement this dish well. Serves 3–5.

2 heaping tablespoons minced fresh ginger
1 heaping tablespoon prepared mustard
1^1/$_2$ teaspoons kelp powder
Juice of 1 lemon
3 tablespoons hempseed oil
14 fluid ounces (1^3/$_4$ cups) coconut milk
4 heaping tablespoons tahini
2 heaping tablespoons hempseed butter
2 pinches cayenne powder

In a small bowl, mix the ginger, mustard, and kelp into the lemon juice and hempseed oil. Stir well. Blend in the coconut milk, again stirring well. Drop the tahini and hempseed butter into the center of the bowl.

Stir well or, for a touch of visual artistry, stir from the center out until an attractive marbled effect is obtained. Sprinkle cayenne on top and serve with salad or as a veggie dip.

Smooth Sesame Sauce

Makes 3¹/₄ cups, enough to cover 4-6 servings of steamed broccoli, winter squash, cooked grains, or pasta.

1¹/₂ cups water
¹/₂ cup toasted sesame butter
1 tablespoon brown rice vinegar
3 tablespoons toasted sesame oil
1 heaping tablespoon kudzu, dissolved in ¹/₄ cup water
¹/₂ garlic bulb, peeled and minced
2 heaping tablespoons minced fresh ginger
¹/₂ teaspoon fenugreek
1 teaspoon whole cumin seeds
1 teaspoon celery seeds
2 heaping tablespoons hempseed flour
1 heaping tablespoon brown rice syrup
6 heaping tablespoons hempseed oil

Bring the water to a boil and add all remaining ingredients (except the hempseed oil). Stir well. When the boil returns, reduce the heat and simmer for 15 minutes. Stir in the hempseed oil just before serving.

Alligator Pear Mash

Serves 2.

> 1 avocado (a.k.a. alligator pear), mashed or cubed, depending on
> ripeness
> $1/2$ garlic bulb, peeled and minced
> Juice of 1 lemon
> 3 tablespoons hempseed oil

Mix all of the ingredients in a bowl. Serve over soba or udon noodles and/or steamed or raw veggies.

DIPS AND SPREADS

If hempseeds had to search out recipes that satisfied all their special needs, I'm sure those with the keenest senses would jump right into dips and spreads. The oil feels safe from free radicals here, because it is not heated in the preparation of these recipes. The milky, mushy, and smooth consistencies are most suitable for facile interfusion of hempseed oil. This is also an appropriate area for exploring the uses of hulled hempseed. See also several dip and spread recipes on pages 75–77 in "Legumes" and Hemp Land and Sea Spread on page 82.

Chillin' Dip

Let's face it, summer is hot! *Why make it any hotter by cooking? You'll also be wise to keep your oil on ice, out of the sun, and all over other delicious live raw foods. On a hot summer day, what could be better than a cool dip? Makes 1 quart.*

    2 cucumbers
    3 cups soy yogurt
    Juice of 1 lemon
    10 tablespoons hempseed oil
    1 handful fresh-picked mint
    $^1/_3$ bunch fresh parsley
    2 cups tahini

With a fork, dig deep lengthwise grooves into the skins of the cukes, all the way around. This will give a stimulating texture. Quarter and slice the cukes into half-bite chunks. Set aside.

Blend all of the remaining ingredients (except the tahini) in an electric blender on high speed. Pour the mixture into a bowl and stir in the tahini, then the reserved cucumber chunks. Serve as dip for veggies, pita, and other breads.

Zuke Ganouj

In my experience, the crop folks most commonly overplant is zucchini. As a result it's the most difficult vegetable to give away. For my home garden, I set a limit of one zucchini mound. Otherwise, I spend many summer nights leaving baskets of zucchini on the doorsteps of my neighbors.

If you fail to harvest zucchini at its prime (it should be small with a deep, dark green color and waxy luster), it will keep growing to the size of your leg. At this size, its flavor has diluted and the flesh has become more watery and airy. Still, I feel these characteristics are worth working with. In this recipe your overgrown zuke performs like an eggplant. Use this creation as you would Baba Ganouj—as a dip or spread for pita bread, naan, chips, or crackers. The yield of this recipe depends largely on the size of your zucchini. Expect to make from 1 to 3 quarts.

1 huge, overgrown zucchini
Extra-virgin olive oil
2 heaping tablespoons tahini
1 tablespoon hempseed butter
3 garlic cloves, peeled and minced
Juice of $^1/_2$ lemon
2 tablespoons hempseed oil
$^1/_2$ teaspoon ground allspice
$^1/_4$ teaspoon ground cumin
2 pinches sea salt
cumin and paprika

Preheat the oven to 425°F (218°C). Peel the zucchini, place it on a cookie sheet, coat with olive oil, and bake for 30 minutes or until the outside has browned. Mash the zuke in a large bowl. Stir in the remaining ingredients. When mixed and mashed completely, let the mixture sit until cool. Before serving, splash a little more hempseed oil on top, then sprinkle on a pinch or two of cumin and paprika.

Wasabi Wakening
Sandwich Spread

Wasabi is a pungent green Oriental horseradish. It is available fresh, powdered, or as a sauce. One must be careful with wasabi because too much ingested at once can be painful. It is a good idea to serve wasabi with a cooling dish on the side such as Chillin' Dip (see page 101). Makes 3 cups.

1 pound tofu, soft or firm
$^1/_2$ cup hempseed oil
Juice of 1 lemon
4 teaspoons wasabi powder (or fresh if available)
2 teaspoons yellow mustard powder
1 teaspoon kelp powder
1 ripe avocado
3 scallions, diced

Mash the tofu well. Form a small well in the center. Into the well add the hempseed oil, then lemon juice, then spices. Stir and mash the mixture. Add the avocado and scallions. Again, stir and mash it well. Spread on a sandwich with lots of sprouts, grated carrot, miso, and cucumber to cool it off.

Sweets:

From Wild Berries
to Decadent Delights

IT'S TIME NOW TO WALK THROUGH THE SWEET PART of the garden. An oasis where we can indulge in both a decadent and healthful way. Hempseed goes as well with sweet foods as with anything else. The special flavor of hempseed complements that of honey, carob, chocolate, dates, fruit, and all kinds of syrups.

Hempify your favorite dessert recipes by substituting hemp milk for dairy milk; hemp butter for nut butters and tahini; hemp flour for a portion of wheat flour; hemp oil for other oils and liquid portions; and sprinkle hulled hempseed over desserts. Here are a handful of original recipes for you to try out.

WILD BERRIES

It's full moon in August or, as I think of it, the Berry Moon. The peak of the season for juicy wild-harvested and cultivated berries here in Cascadia. From the wild come salmonberries, strawberries, huckleberries, raspberries, blackberries, salal, and thimbleberries. Cascadians tend to grow a highbush blueberry that yields huge, juicy fruits. Areas of the Northwest are rapidly gaining respect as fantastic wine regions.

The relationship between people and the naturalized Himalayan blackberry drastically changes toward the middle of the summer. Folks lay down their shears, machetes, and herbicidal tendencies to pick up their baskets, ladders, and pie pans. Like cannabis, blackberry is one plant that has many extraordinary characteristics. It perseveringly grows fast and deep to take back the earth from concrete, asphalt, and human messes; to cleanse, nourish, and stabilize the soil it grows in; and feed us critters, too. See what full-moon berry magic you can whip up using your own local berries.

Berry Moon Raw Fruit Pie

Serves 8.

 ¹/₂ cup almonds
 4 cups dates
 1 cup fresh figs
 ¹/₂ cup sunflower seeds, hulled
 ¹/₂ cup hempseed flour
 1 cup oats
 2 peaches
 3 plums
 3 cups any combination of juicy, locally harvested fresh berries
 2 bananas
 ¹/₂ cup hempseed oil

To make the crust, grind the almonds in a hand-cranked grinder with large holes. Pit the dates and stem the figs. Combine the almonds, dates, and figs with the sunflower seeds, flour, and oats in a large bowl and mash well. Press this into the sides of an 8-inch or larger pie pan to form a mold.

To make the filling, slice and pit the remainder of the fruit, and stir it up with the hempseed oil. Scoop and spread inside the crust. Remember, this is a *raw* fruit pie, so don't be throwing it in the oven. It's cool and it's done. Enjoy!

Blueberry Nut Syrup

Serves 4-6.

Delicious over pancakes (see recipes on pages 124 and 125).

- $^1/_4$ cup maple syrup
- 1 cup molasses
- 3 heaping tablespoons hempseed butter
- 2 cups blueberries, frozen, canned, or fresh
- $^1/_2$ cup walnuts, chopped
- $^1/_2$ cup pecans, chopped

Heat the syrup and molasses in an iron saucepan over high heat until the mixture begins to foam. Remove from the heat until foam subsides. Place back onto medium heat. Add the remaining ingredients. Increase the heat to medium-high and cook for another 5 minutes. Serve while hot, but cooling.

Vegan Hemp
Raspberry Cheese Cake

Paul Benhaim, formerly the managing director of New Earth Ltd., can often be found cruising neighborhoods and events in a hemp ice cream van serving sweet frozen hempseed delights. This is a project of the Hemp Food Industries Association to promote hemp foods. Paul has also shared this great dessert recipe with us. Makes one 8-inch pie.

2 cups crushed digestive biscuits (low-fat vegan)*
$^3/_4$ cup hempseed flour
$^1/_2$ stick (4 tablespoons) organic, nonhydrogenated margarine
1 pound silken tofu
3 tablespoons golden syrup*
$^1/_2$ cup raw cane sugar
Juice of 1 lemon
Pinch sea salt
2 teaspoons vanilla extract
2 large bananas
$^1/_2$ pound fresh raspberries

To make the crust, mix the biscuits, hempseed flour, and margarine in a food processor until they're combined. Pat the mixture into an 8-inch round pie tin; cover and refrigerate until you're ready for it.

Preheat the oven to 350°F (177°C). Whisk together all the remaining ingredients until they're well mixed. Pour into the pie shell and bake for 35 to 40 minutes, or until firm.

*Digestive biscuits and Tate and Lyle's Golden Syrup are ingredients fancied throughout England but are available to Americans only in specialty food stores in larger cities. To substitute for digestive biscuits, try graham crackers, sweet granola, or broken-up crunchy cookies. For the golden syrup, substitute high-quality cane syrup or light honey.

Hemp-Berry Filling

Makes two 8-inch-round pies.

> 4 cups fresh or frozen berries of your choice
> $^1/_2$ cup hempseed butter
> 2 cups honey

If berries are frozen, defrost them in a mixing bowl. Add the rest of the ingredients and stir gently until consistent. Follow instructions for Hempy Pie Crust (page 116). I prefer this pie with a top crust.

SWEET AND CITRUS FRUITS

Wherever you go in this world, you will find the blessings of the earth's sweetness in the form of a fruit particular to that region. It could be the mango of the Tropics, Georgia peaches, Florida oranges, northwestern plums, Central American bananas, island coconuts, or California dates. I've never met a fruit that didn't go well with hempseed.

Most fruits love to be bathed in and mashed with hempseed oil.

Hempseed Yogurt Fruit Salad

For the fruits listed in this recipe, you are free to substitute whatever is in season, available, and regionally grown. Serves 2.

2 cups soy yogurt
1 heaping tablespoon fruit jam of your choice
¹/₄ cup hempseed oil
1 heaping tablespoon bee pollen
1 mango, sliced thin or mushed, depending on ripeness
1 apple, cut into bite-sized wedges
1 navel orange, peeled and wedged
2 bananas, sliced into bite-sized pieces
1 cup in-season berries

Combine the soy yogurt, jam, hempseed oil, and bee pollen. Stir well until smooth. Stir in the fruits and serve.

Hempseed Freeze

Makes ¹/₂ gallon.

> 14 fluid ounces (1³/₄ cups) coconut milk
> 1 cup hempseed butter
> 3 tablespoons hempseed oil
> ¹/₃ cup barley malt
> About 8 ripe bananas

Combine the coconut milk, hempseed butter, hempseed oil, and barley malt in a blender or food processor and blend at high speed. Add the bananas one at a time until the mixture is about as thick as the machine will allow. Blend for another minute. Serve some immediately as a thick shake and/or place in a container and freeze to achieve an ice-cream-like consistency.

Cool California Topping

This makes a great topping for desserts. Makes $^1/_2$ gallon.

    2 cups dates
    2 cups fresh figs
    2 bananas
    1 softball-sized mango
    $^1/_4$ cup hempseed oil

Stem the figs, pit the dates, peel and chop the bananas, and peel and pit the mango. Combine in a large bowl with the hempseed oil. Mash well for 5 minutes and serve.

Hemp Nutty Cookies

Makes 2 dozen.

1¹/₂ cups whole wheat flour
1 cup rolled oats
1 cup hulled hempseed
2 tablespoons freshly ground flaxseed meal
¹/₂ teaspoon sea salt
1 teaspoon baking powder
³/₄ cup safflower oil
¹/₂ cup honey
¹/₂ cup warm water
¹/₄ cup sliced brazil nuts
¹/₄ cup chopped walnuts

Preheat oven to 375°F (190°C). Combine flour, oats, hulled hempseed, flax meal, salt, and baking powder in a mixing bowl. Stir well, then form a well at the center. Pour oil into the well and stir it in. Dissolve the honey in the water, then stir it into the mixture until consistent. The batter should be moist and thick. Now stir in the nuts.

Drop heaping tablespoons of batter onto ungreased cookie sheets and bake 10 to 15 minutes, until brown.

Seedy Sweeties

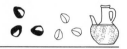

Seedy Sweeties were the main product my company, Hungry Bear Hemp Foods, produced and distributed throughout North America. Being the second hemp food product to come out on the market, this was the first taste of hempseed for thousands of people. As they were loved and appreciated by many, I received countless requests for the recipe, which I politely declined. Now that they are no longer being produced, I can withhold the recipe no longer. Makes 2-3 11 x 17-inch cookie sheets.

1^1/$_3$ cups sweet Barbados molasses

^{2}/$_3$ cup brown rice syrup

Or replace the above two syrups with 2 cups pure sorghum syrup
    if available.

2 cups whole or hulled hempseed

2 cups oat flour

2^1/$_3$ cups brown sesame seed

1^1/$_3$ cups cashews (for nutty type), or sunflower seeds (for sunflower
    type)

1 cup Brazil nuts (for nutty type), or sunflower seeds (for sunflower
    type)

Hempseed oil

Oil your cookie sheets with hempseed oil.

Combine the hempseed, oat flour, 1^1/$_3$ cups of the sesame seed, and the cashews (or sunflower seeds) in a wok or large, sturdy mixing bowl.

In a large saucepan heat syrups at high heat. Insert candy thermometer so that the tip is submerged in the syrup, but not touching the pan. After a few minutes the syrups will begin to foam up. When this occurs, turn the heat down until the foam subsides, being careful not to get splattered. Return to high heat and partially cover. Check the temperature often. When the syrups reach 270°F (132°C) (the temperature can be varied from between 250°F [121°C] [soft] to 300°F [149°C] [hard] depending on your preferred hardness) remove from heat and immediately pour into the seed mix. Stir until consistent.

Quickly pour onto the oiled cookie sheets. Spread mixture as evenly as you can, then roll flat with a rolling pin oiled with hempseed oil. If it gets sticky, just allow to cool for a few minutes then try again. After fifteen minutes, cut into squares with a pizza cutter.

Combine the rest of the sesame seeds with the Brazil nuts (or sunflower seeds) and run the mixture through a steel hand-cranked food grinder with the medium-sized-hole plate. This will grind them into a coarse, oily meal.

When the treats are cool enough to work with, scrape each square from the cookie sheet, roll each in the ground seed, and serve. If you have difficulty removing treats from pans, warm the bottom of the pan.

Hempy Pie Crust

Makes two 8-inch bottoms and two tops—or three bottoms and no tops.

 1 cup hulled hempseed
 $^1/_3$ cup Brazil nuts, ground into a meal
 $^1/_3$ cup walnuts, ground into a meal
 $^1/_3$ cup flaxseed meal
 1 cup whole wheat flour
 1 cup rolled oats
 1 teaspoon sea salt
 $1^1/_4$ cups safflower oil
 1 cup hempseed oil
 $^1/_2$ cup water

Preheat oven to 375°F (190°C). Combine all ingredients in a mixing bowl and stir well. For double-crust pies, press half of the mixture into the bottoms of two 8-inch-round pie tins, making the crust about $^1/_4$ inch thick. Bake for 5 to 7 minutes, until crust has browned slightly. Fill with your favorite filling. To make the top crust, roll out remaining mixture to $^1/_4$ inch thick and lay on top of filling in whatever pattern you wish. Bake again for 20 to 25 minutes, until crust browns. If you prefer single-crust pies, divide the mixture evenly among three 8-inch pie tins. Allow to cool before serving.

Winter Squash Pie Filling

Makes two 8-inch pies.

4 cups cooked squash meat (any type of winter squash or pumpkin will
    work)
$^1/_2$ cup hempseed butter
2 cups honey

Combine all ingredients in a bowl and stir well. Follow instructions for Hempy Pie
Crust on page 116. I prefer this pie without a top crust.

Hemp Smudge

What you do with this fudge—Silly Putty hybrid is up to you. The standard approach would be to roll it up, but I have a feeling the Hemp Smudge fairy will evoke the Silly Putty sculptor in you! Makes ¹/₂ cup.

   4 heaping tablespoons barley malt
   1 tablespoon carob powder
   3 heaping tablespoons hempseed butter

Heat the barley malt in a small iron skillet over medium-high heat. When the malt begins to boil, add the remaining ingredients. Increase the heat to high and stir well for a few minutes. Let cool.

   The mixture will cool down to Tootsie Roll–like consistency. Have fun with it! Mush it, knead it, spread it, or fold it over. Isn't it great that it doesn't stick to the pan?

Alien Nut
Polka-Dot Spread

Makes 2 1/2 cups.

- 1/2 cup tahini
- 1/4 cup hempseed butter
- 1/2 cup almond butter
- 1 ripe avocado
- 1/4 cup fruit jam of your choice
- 2 tablespoons maple syrup
- 2 heaping tablespoons bee pollen
- 1 tablespoon spirulina or blue-green algae powder
- 1/4 cup hempseed oil

Just stir everything together well, spread on rice cakes or other sweet cakes, and enjoy!

Baking with Hempseed

IN ADDITION TO THE DESSERT RECIPES in the preceding chapter, both hempseed flour and hulled hempseed are worthwhile additions to just about any baked goods recipe, from yeasted breads to quick breads and muffins. Hempseed makes a great addition to pancakes as well. I've included some of my favorites here and with a simple rule of thumb you can adapt any baked good recipe to include hemp.

The most common ingredient in baked goods is wheat flour. This is because wheat has the highest content of the proteins glutenin and gliadin, which form gluten when combined with water. Gluten is what makes the dough spongy and elastic, and holds it all together (*gluten* is Latin for "glue"). As far as I know, hempseed has little or none of the proteins that compose gluten, therefore using hempseed as your sole flour ingredient will not produce bread as you know it. Other grains high in the proteins that compose gluten are rye and spelt.

Here are the rules of thumb that I apply to most baked good recipes:

1. For leavened breads, combine up to 1 part hempseed flour (or hulled hempseed) with 2 parts glutenous flours.
2. For quick breads, combine up to 1 part hempseed flour (or hulled hempseed) with 1 part other flours.

LEAVENED BREAD

As there is as much to say about bread making as there is about hemp food-crafting, I prefer to refer you elsewhere to learn the fine craft of bread making. The two books I most recommend are *The Tassajara Bread Book* and *The Laurel's Kitchen Bread Book* (see appendix 2, "Suggested Reading"). These books teach two unique methods for making and appreciating whole-grain breads.

The addition of a tablespoon or two of hempseed oil makes a "cakier" bread and adds that special nutty, rich flavor. Using oil-rich hulled hempseed will achieve this too as well as adding bits of hempseed kernel to the texture of the crust and interior.

Hemp Beer Bread

The Frederick Brewing Company of Frederick, Maryland, brews up
Hempen Ale and Hempen Gold beers and shares this beer bread
recipe (see appendix 1 for sources of hemp beer). Makes 1 loaf.

3$^1/_2$ cups all-purpose flour

$^1/_4$ cup sugar

1 teaspoon salt

1 teaspoon baking soda

1 teaspoon baking powder

1 bottle (12 ounces) Hempen Ale, at room temperature

1 egg

Preheat the oven to 350°F (177°F). Mix the flour, sugar, salt, baking soda, and baking powder. Add the Hempen Ale and egg; mix well. Pour into a greased, standard loaf pan and bake for approximately 50 minutes.

Huggin' Muffins

Let's put some love in that oven! Makes 2¹/₂ dozen muffins.

1¹/₂ cups hempseed flour
1¹/₂ cups rice flour
1¹/₂ cups cornmeal
1¹/₂ cups whole wheat pastry flour
1¹/₂ teaspoons baking powder
1 cup brown rice syrup
¹/₄ cup safflower oil
1 teaspoon kudzu dissolved in 1 cup water
Ricemilk or hempmilk (Have 2 cups on hand, you may not need all of it.)

Preheat the oven to 375°F (190°C). In a large bowl, mix together the dry ingredients. Stir in the brown rice syrup, oil, and kudzu-water mix. Slowly stir in ricemilk or hempmilk until the mixture is thick with no dry spots—then stop stirring (too much stirring doesn't help). Oil muffin tins and fill them with batter almost all the way to the top. Bake for 30 minutes. Remove from tins and allow to cool.

Hemp and Whole Wheat Pancakes

Serves 4-6.

1^1/$_2$ cups hempseed flour
1^1/$_2$ cups whole wheat flour
1^1/$_2$ heaping tablespoons turbinado sugar
1 tablespoon baking powder
1 teaspoon sea salt
3 tablespoons hempseed oil
3 cups water
Safflower oil

In a large bowl, combine all the ingredients (except the safflower oil) in order. Oil an iron skillet with safflower oil and heat it over a medium-high flame. Using a ladle or pitcher, drop the mixture onto the skillet into palm-sized round cakes. Peek under each cake. When they turn that golden-brown color, it is time to flip. Cook only once on each side. Serve topped with fruit, yogurt, and/or Blueberry Nut Syrup (page 107).

Wheat-Free
Hemp Pancakes

Serves 6–8.

2 cups hempseed flour
1 cup corn flour
1 cup oat flour
1 cup brown rice flour
3 heaping tablespoons turbinado sugar
5 teaspoons baking powder
1 teaspoon sea salt
6 tablespoons hempseed oil
5 cups water
Safflower oil

In a large bowl, combine all the ingredients (except the safflower oil) in order. Oil an iron skillet with safflower oil and heat it over a medium-high flame. Using a ladle or pitcher, drop the mixture onto the skillet into palm-sized round cakes. Peek under each cake. When they turn that golden-brown color, it is time to flip. Cook only once on each side. Serve topped with fruit, yogurt, and/or Blueberry Nut Syrup (page 107).

A Sip of Hemp

To complement your hemp food cuisine, there are a variety of hemp beverages available. Nondairy hempmilk is one that you can make in your own kitchen, to be used for drinking or cooking. And you'll find several varieties of hemp coffee, beer, and wine produced commercially (also see appendix 1 for sources of these products).

HEMPMILK

Hempmilk is one of the most enjoyable, versatile, and satisfying ways to enjoy hempseed. One of the bestselling categories of items on the natural food market are nondairy beverages. Due to objections by the dairy industry, nondairy beverages cannot be marketed as "milk." However, I am not marketing anything, and nondairy liquids are included in the definition of milk so I reserve my right to use that term. Milks made from soybeans, rice, almonds, and grains are favorites of vegans to use in just about any way that one would use cow's milk.

Unfortunately, all of the nondairy milks are available only in drink boxes. Although it offers an extremely long shelf life, the packaging is excessive, toxic, and difficult to recycle. People who live eco-conscious lifestyles and love nondairy milk are stuck in this eco-consumerist dilemma. A couple of friends of mine came up with a solution by starting a company that produced fresh soymilk, packaged it in recycled glass bottles, and made deliveries by bicycle.

An even better solution is to make it yourself at home with hempseed as your main ingredient. When I produced hempmilk (in recycled glass bottles) for local Eugene natural food stores, my customers would often exclaim how the taste is as good or better than popular soymilk brands and how good it makes their bodies feel. I found myself doing something unheard of in the business world by teaching my best customers how to make my product at home.

Hempmilk is easy to make at home provided you have the necessary tools: a Champion Juicer (or similar model) with a large-holed screen, a funnel, and cheesecloth. You can use it just about any way that you would use cow's milk—straight, in breakfast cereal, recipes, coffee drinks, shakes, and smoothies. Its easy to hempify baked goods recipes by substituting hempmilk for water.

To make hempmilk, use the basic hempmilk instructions for any of my favorite hempmilk variations that follow. Once you have mastered the process you can create your own variations by substituting different grains, beans, nuts, sweeteners, and flavorings.

If you still like to drink from a box, HempNut Incorporated may soon produce hempmilk in the aseptic drink box.

Basic Hempmilk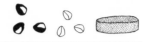

Makes 1 quart.

Water
1 cup hempseed (whole, cake, or hulled)
1 to 4 tablespoons honey (optional)

Soak the hempseed (with grains, nuts, or seeds if called for by the recipe) overnight in a jar filled with water with a loosely fitting lid. Strain the seed and save the soaking water.

Heat a quart of water (including the soaking water) in a saucepan to 130° to 140°F (55° to 60°C). Set up your Champion juicer with a large-holed screen installed, a medium-sized bowl under the screen, and a large bowl under the end of the hub to catch the meal (see photo 1).

Pour the soaked seed into the funnel $^{1}/_{2}$ cup at a time. Pour just enough hot water into the funnel to keep the seed submerged and push down firmly (push gently if using hulled hempseed) with the plunger (see photo 2). Alternate water and plunger pressure until all the seed has gone through the machine. The hempmilk concentrate will fall from the screen into the bowl beneath. When the bowl gets full, pour its contents into a clean quart bottle (with a tight-fitting lid) through a funnel lined with cheesecloth or a strainer to filter out particles (see photo 3). Repeat until the soaked seed is used up.

If the machine stalls, you may be pressing too hard, not adding enough water, or have a dull cutter in your juicer. If the meal appears whitish, run it through the machine once more. Keep running hulled hempseed through the machine until the full quart is produced.

Add the sweetener and flavorings to the hempmilk concentrate in the bottle. Run some more hot water through the machine and use it to fill the rest of the bottle. Shake it up, chill, and enjoy! Natural separation will occur, so shake it up before use. This will last a few days refrigerated. Everyone has a unique sweet tooth, so the recipes call for 1 to 4 tablespoons of sweetener per quart.

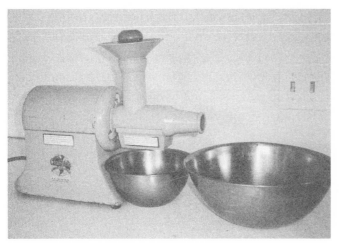

1. Champion juicer and bowls ready for making hempmilk.

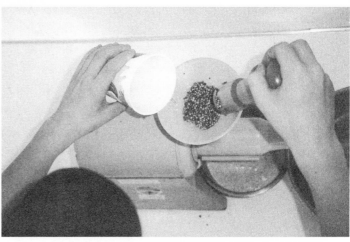

2. Pouring water over hempseed in funnel and pushing with plunger.

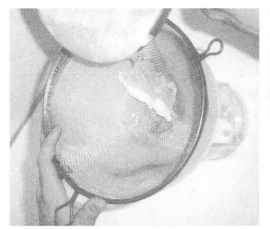

3. Pouring hempmilk concentrate through strainer to filter out particles.

The following two recipes are products called CannaBeverage, which I produced for Eugene's natural food stores. The sesame seed and oats add a thick body and creamy texture. The sesame seed also provides over 140 mg of calcium per 8 fluid ounce serving—that's over 20 percent of the U.S. RDA for an adult. To enrich this recipe with vitamin D, expose your skin to direct sunlight while drinking hempmilk.

Vanilla Hempmilk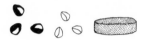

Follow instructions on page 128. Makes one quart.

Water
$^1/_3$ cup hempseed (whole, cake, or hulled)
$^1/_3$ cup sesame seed, whole, brown
$^1/_3$ cup oats (rolled, quick, or steel cut)
1 to 4 tablespoons honey
$^1/_2$ teaspoon vanilla extract

Chocolate Hempmilk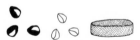

Follow instructions on page 128. Makes 1 quart.

Water
$^1/_3$ cup hempseed (whole, cake, or hulled)
$^1/_3$ cup sesame seed, whole, brown
$^1/_3$ cup oats (rolled, quick, or steel cut)
1 to 4 tablespoons honey
$^1/_4$ cup chocolate syrup

Add the chocolate syrup when combining all the liquids. Shake it well.

Maple-Almond Hempmilk

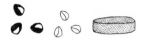

Follow instructions on page 128. Makes 1 quart.

- $^1/_3$ cup hempseed (whole, cake, or hulled)
- $^1/_3$ cup almonds
- $^1/_3$ cup oats (rolled or steel cut)
- 1 to 4 tablespoons maple syrup
- $^1/_2$ teaspoon almond extract

Hempseed-Almond-Sunflower Milk

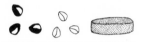

Follow instructions on page 128. Makes 1 quart.

- $^1/_3$ cup hempseed (whole, cake, or hulled)
- $^1/_3$ cup almonds
- $^1/_3$ cup sunflower kernels
- 1 to 4 tablespoons honey or brown rice syrup
- $^1/_2$ teaspoon vanilla extract

Soak hempseed, almonds, and sunflower kernels together. Consume this within a day, as sunflower kernels turn quickly in liquid form.

Carob-Mint Hempmilk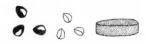

Follow instructions on page 128. Makes 1 quart.

Water
$^1/_3$ cup hempseed (whole, cake, or hulled)
$^1/_3$ cup sesame seed, whole, brown
$^1/_3$ cup oats (rolled, quick, or steel cut)
2 tablespoons toasted carob powder
1 to 4 tablespoons honey
$^1/_2$ teaspoon peppermint extract

Add the carob powder while combining the liquid ingredients. Shake well!

Sweet Sorghum Hempmilk

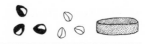

Like hemp, sorghum is a food, fiber, and fuel crop. The grain is very similar to corn and is used to make masa, flour, and animal feed. The tall stalk is used for fiber, firewood, and ethanol production. Sweet sorghum syrup is extracted from the cane and cooked down for over a day. Sorghum used to be a big crop in the southeastern United States. It is still grown widely for animal feed. Sorghum syrup production has been reduced to a cottage industry. Sorghum festivals are still held in northern Georgia.

Most syrups marketed as sorghum by big companies are actually corn syrup with a small amount of sorghum. You are best off finding a brand made by a small family farm with a label that says "100% pure sorghum syrup." Follow instructions for basic hempmilk on page 128. Makes 1 quart.

Water
2 cups hempseed (whole, cake, or hulled)
2 cups sesame seed, whole, brown
2 cups oats (rolled, quick, or steel cut)
$1/4$ cup sweet sorghum syrup

If sorghum syrup is nowhere to be found, a combination of 3 tablespoons sweet Barbados molasses and 1 tablespoon brown rice syrup makes a fine substitute.

Steamed Hempmilk

Starting with the recipes above for hempmilk, you can make any of the popular coffee drinks with steamed hempmilk. It would be appropriate to use a hempseed-coffee blend (see page 138). Makes nearly 1 cup.

> 1/2 cup hempseed milk
> 2 heaping tablespoons raw cane sugar

Combine ingredients in a steaming cup. Insert the stem of your steamer and steam until foam stops rising. Serve immediately on top of your favorite coffee drink.

Cannabis Chai

French-type press pots are the preferred steeping vessel for this and other hot hempseed flour beverage recipes. Be sure to stir just before pressing. Add maple syrup to taste (optional). Don't have a press pot? Then just use a teapot and filter it through some hemp summer cloth. Makes 2 cups.

- 2 heaping tablespoons hempseed flour
- 1 teaspoon stevia powder
- 1 teaspoon carob powder
- $1/2$ teaspoon ground cinnamon
- 6 cardamom pods
- 1 whole star of star anise
- $1/4$ teaspoon fennel seed
- $1/4$ teaspoon whole coriander seed
- $1/4$ teaspoon ground nutmeg
- Pinch freshly ground black pepper
- 3 dime-sized pieces of orange peel, fresh or dried
- 6 dime-sized pieces of fresh ginger, peeled
- $2 1/2$ cups boiling water
- Maple syrup (optional)

Mix the first 10 ingredients a small bowl until consistent. Pour into your steeping vessel of choice along with the orange peel and ginger. Add the boiling water. Steep for 15 minutes, stirring every few minutes.

If you are wondering where the sweetener is in this recipe, it's the stevia, anise, and fennel. Just as the cannabis plant has the potential to replace the wood fiber, petrochemical, and cotton industries, so these herbs (particularly stevia) are healthful alternatives to white sugar, saccharin, and artificial sweeteners. Combining such plants increases the nourishing and liberating powers of food—and in turn empowers those who drink it!

Hemp Nog

The snow may blow, the flu may flow, but Hemp Nog will keep you healthy! The recipe I share with you for winter solstice encompasses the distinguishing qualities of this time of year: sharing, caring, feasting, and keeping healthy. This recipe is a carefully formulated herbal-medicinal concoction for warmth, decongestion, improved circulation, and an enhanced immune system. Makes 1 quart.

3$^1/_2$ cups water
2 heaping tablespoons cardamom pods
2 teaspoons fennel seeds
1 heaping teaspoon whole cloves
2 pinches black pepper
2 heaping tablespoons tapioca
$^1/_2$ teaspoon kudzu
1 teaspoon ground cinnamon
$^1/_2$ teaspoon ground nutmeg
$^1/_4$ cup hempseed oil
$^1/_2$ cup brown rice syrup
1 cup hempseed flour

To make the tea, bring 1$^3/_4$ cups of the water to a boil. Turn off the heat. Steep the following spices for 20 minutes: cardamom, fennel, cloves, and black pepper. Strain.

To make the starch broth, add the tapioca and kudzu to 1$^3/_4$ cups of water in a saucepan and whisk gently. Let sit for 5 minutes.

Add the tea to the starch broth, then add the cinnamon and nutmeg. Bring to a boil, reduce the heat, and simmer for 10 minutes. Whisk gently. Add the hempseed oil, then the brown rice syrup. (*Hint:* If you use the same measuring cup for both liquids without washing it, the syrup will not stick to the sides of the measuring cup, thanks to hempseed oil lubrication.) Add the hempseed flour. Stir until consistent. Cover and set aside for 20 minutes. Stir well. Blend in an electric blender on high speed for a minute, a couple of cups at a time. Pour into a bottle and set it in the fridge undisturbed for 3 hours, allowing the particles to settle. Then, without shaking, pour it into a serving container, leaving the settled particles behind. Serve warm or cold. Add rum to taste if that's your thing.

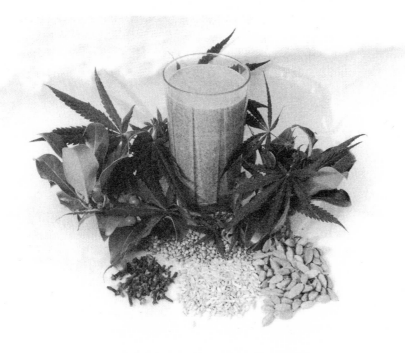

Hempnog—a drink both festive and healthy.

JAVA CANNABISSA!

Wandering through a northwestern city you'd be surprised to find a single street corner void of its coffeeshop or espresso stand. Although caffeine has so rapidly become the drug of choice for working Americans, hemp coffee producers fortunately have not capitalized on that talked-about "drug appeal" of hemp products. Rather, they have focused their efforts on making and marketing quality coffee blends.

Hempfields Natural Goods hit the market first with three blends formulated for different times of the day: Hemprising (morning), 420 Blend (you know when), and HempXpress (midnight oil). The Galaxy Global Eatery in New York City markets its own blend of Sumatran Sunrise Vanilla Hemp.

The only whole-bean/whole-seed hemp coffee blend available is called Sumativa from Humboldt Hemp Foods. Whole-bean/whole-seed coffee has the advantage of maintaining its fresh taste for you to crack open when you grind it before brewing.

All the above products are excellent blends. Unless you live in the above locales, however, the freshness will to some degree deteriorate over the time the coffee spends in transit and shelf sitting. To ensure the freshest hemp coffee, you must start with your choice of freshly roasted coffee beans and add whole hempseed that you have freshly roasted. A ratio of about 1 heaping tablespoon of hempseed to 1 cup of coffee beans should work fine. Grind together and prepare as you normally would make a pot of coffee.

While our minds are in high gear, let's direct some cogitation toward the possible ill effects of coffee abuse, to help us determine our own limits of responsible use. First off, coffee doesn't *give* us energy. It actually triggers the release of epinephrine (adrenaline), which our body usually produces for emergency use only.

In grade school there were kids who used to pull fire alarms for kicks. They knew they were doing a service—keeping the principals and teachers on their toes. To an extent I still feel that way! At any rate, if they had pulled the alarms every day, the excitement would have dwindled, people would've begun failing to respond, and major adult irritation would have resulted.

The point is that we do not want to put our bodies through a fire drill every day. Too much caffeine can overtax our adrenal glands, tweak our nervous systems, and cause fatigue over the long term.

Coffee may also cause frequent urination, thereby overworking our kidneys. If we fail to replenish our bodies with water, we might suffer the effects of dehydration. When I drink coffee, I fill a glass of the same size with water and make sure to drink both at the same rate. A gulp of cool, clear water helps wash me out of that hole, replenishes my thirsty cells, and flows me back into the ocean of earth energy.

Anyway, didn't mean to ruin your buzz. If you are alert to the effects that coffee drinking has on your energy level, habits, and overall health, then you're likely to stay within your limits of healthy coffee drinking. I must admit that much of this book was written late at night, high on caffeine. See appendix 1 for mail-order distributors of hemp coffee.

CHEERS! WITH HEMP BEER

The most recent place in our social lives that we can find cannabis is on tap at the local pub. Yes, many microbreweries in North America and Europe have found that hempseed makes a fantastic ingredient in beer. Hempseed is not just a novelty ingredient to attract attention; it offers a unique flavor and finish, and is more mellow and less bitter than hops. Brewmeisters use hempseed meal as a direct substitution for up to one-third of their hops.

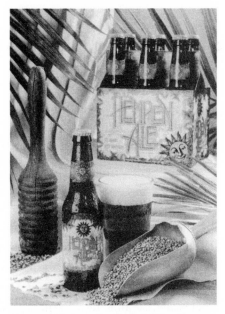

Hempen Ale from the Frederick Brewing Company.

In fact, cannabis is a close relative of hops (genus *Humulus* in the hemp family Cannabinaceae). So close, in fact, that you can actually graft a cannabis stem onto a hop vine; it will mature and flower!

Hempen Ale from the Frederick Brewing Company is the winner of many prestigious awards, including a bronze medal for brewing excellence in the herb/spice category at the 16th Great American Beer Festival, the most highly regarded beer event in the United States. In 1997 the company began offering a cream ale called Hempen Gold.

This well-accepted modern-day beer tradition continues with another hemp ale produced by the Humboldt Brewing Company and Kentucky Hemp Beer, from the Limestone Brewing Company. See appendix 1 for addresses of hemp beer suppliers.

I'm excited to see what tasty concoctions will come from the fermentations of home brewers!

HEMP WINE

What would be a more appropriate beverage to accompany fine cannabis cuisine than a bottle of hemp wine? From Hemp Wine America in the Finger Lakes region comes a fine white wine blended with natural hemp. Formulated from seed-pressed extract (essential oil of hempseed), this is a semisweet white wine that has a burst of initial flavor and an incredibly strong finish. Although most white wines are served chilled, this one is best served at room temperature to make the hemp flavor stand out more.

Hemp Wine America is licensed to produce this wine by Nirvana Homebrews, which is the Dutch company that came up with the process for extracting the essential seed oil and formulating it in wine. As of this printing, these are the only companies in the world that produce hemp wine. HWA has recently introduced a red wine. See appendix 1 for the address of Hemp Wine America.

PART 3

Further Tales of Hempseed

Food for Feathers, Fins, and Four Legs

HUMANS ARE PROBABLY JUST ONE of the more recent species on this planet to discover the delicious hempseed. Birds fed on wild cannabis for ages before human civilization took shape. As agriculture evolved, hemp fields rapidly became an important part of the diet of wild birds migrating in autumn.

The move to prohibit hemp farming and the resultant growth of timber, cotton, petrochemical, and pharmaceutical industries have caused incalculable harm to the ecology and wildlife of our beautiful home planet. The migrating bird populations that once depended on the abundance of the hemp fields of the Midwest have been forced to rely upon wild hemp for their hempfood supply.

The U.S. government later set out to rid the continent of cannabis by launching extensive eradication projects (mass sprayings of herbicides). The plants that do survive this senseless act of biocide are often contaminated with toxic residues. The poisons are passed from the birds that eat the tainted seeds to their chicks as well as to the animals higher on the food chain.

Even domesticated birds had much to lose from prohibition. In 1937 birdseed companies pleaded with Congress to allow the importation of sterilized hempseed. "The songbirds won't sing without it," they affirmed in their testimony. If not for these lobbying efforts, hempseed of any type would probably not be legally available in the United States for birds or humans.

Hempseed is a favorite among many varieties of wild, exotic, and songbirds. It helps the birds maintain a healthy immune system and shiny, lustrous feathers.

A Kentucky cattle farmer, Donnie Coulter, has been conducting a pilot experiment by supplementing the feed for his beef cattle with hempseed. He is using hempseed meal he obtained from a brewery that couldn't use it because it was ground too fine.[1] The supplement has resulted in happier, shinier, and more energetic animals. At auction, the hemp-fed cattle sold for three cents more per pound than non-hemp-fed cows.[2]

Convinced by the results, Coulter is now marketing the meal under the name Nutrahemp by Circle C Farm Enterprises. It comes as a fine-ground meal or in lumps with a discount for those who help with research documentation.[3]

Vegetarian hemp-burgers have been served by many hemp food vendors to promote alternatives to beef. However, the hemp-burgers served up by the White Light Diner in Frankfort, Kentucky, are made of the beef raised by Coulter. The first beef hemp-burgers were served in May 1998. Many customers were impressed with the taste and concept, while others were unable to tell the difference.[4]

The real results will be evident in the health of the cows. If the EFAs benefit the cows' immune systems, antibiotic use may decrease. If hempseed's protein effectuates faster weight gain, the use of growth hormones may ease. This would be good news for the health of meat eaters as well as the economics of cattle farming (of course, the health of both meat eaters and cows would be further enhanced by going vegetarian). Hempseed has also been prescribed as a laxative for constipated farm animals for several hundred years in both Europe and Asia.

Aquaculture investigators at Kentucky State University have been feeding blue catfish a mixture of hempseed meal, vitamins, minerals, and fatty acids. LNA is an essential nutrient in the fish diet, but unlike humans fish can convert LA from LNA, so they don't require LA in their diet.[5] The fish seemed to like the hempseed and grew at a normal rate even with a simple bare nutrient diet.[6] Perchance their ancestors fed on hempseed that made its way into the streams and rivers during Kentucky's hemp-farming heyday. Perhaps a hemp-farming revival would be a blessing to myriad native fish species.

Hempseed is sold at bait stores in Europe. Anglers find it one of the most effective baits for chumming in fresh water.[7]

As for any of the fish and animals that are farmed commercially, cost is often the bottom line. While the prices of domestic soybeans and cottonseed (major feed ingredients for most farmed animals and fish) remain but a fraction of the price of imported hempseed (meal), only those farmers who honor the sublimity of hempseed will use it in quantity.

The dogs and cats we love so dearly can benefit from the hempseed as well. My cats go crazy when I pour hempseed oil over their dry food. The taste is reminiscent of seafood. When my dogs are good, they are treated to hemp dog biscuits.

Free to Pee THC

Recently we have come to learn that a positive urine analysis for THC may result after consuming hempseed. The springboard issue occurred back in late August of 1996 when Aegis Laboratories, a forensic lab in Tennessee, made public its plea to the DEA and FDA to have my main product, Seedy Sweeties, removed from the market, because it exposes the inaccuracies of their tests. The FDA and DEA studied the lab's claim and held that hempseeds contain no illegal levels of THC, are legal import products, and have been cleared for culinary use.[1, 2, 3]

In December 1997 Air Force Master Sergeant Spencer Gaines was acquitted in a court-martial after showing that his consumption of hempseed oil caused him to test positive. Five months later a jury overturned the court-martial of Lance Corporal Kevin Boyd, who had been accused of smoking marijuana.[4]

All of these events prompted the drug-testing industry to pressure Congress into rash actions, such as banning hemp products from the market.

Recent studies conducted by Dr. J. C. Callaway confirm that traces of cannabinoid metabolites can be detected in the urine within hours after consuming hempseed oil.[5] The results show that you can test positive whether you consume hempseed oil every day or up to twenty-nine hours after a one-time ingestion.[6] (See an article by Dr. Callaway and his associates reprinted at the end of this chapter.)

Further investigation revealed that edible hempseed is far from being the only factor that reveals the inaccuracy of urine testing. For instance, the following anti-inflammatory drugs (phenylpropionic acid derivatives) produce positive cannabinoid results in screen tests: ibuprofen (Motrin; Advil), naproxin (Anaprox; Naprosyn), and fenoprofen (Nalfon).[7] Also, as this $600-million-a-year industry continues to grow, so does the quantity of specimens analyzed—increasing the likelihood of human error.

In most cases, urine tests are performed using a combination of two types of tests. The first test is a *screen test*, usually an immunoassay; it indicates whether the target chemical compound binds to an antibody. This is a very inexpensive test to perform, and labs are often automated to perform a large number of tests rapidly. It does not give an accurate level of the substance tested for, only a simple "positive" or "negative." In the case of THC testing, labs usually test for the metabolite 11-nor-9-tetrahydrocannabinol-9-carboxylic acid (THC-COOH), which also cross-reacts with other cannabinoids. Because the screen test lacks an acceptable level of accuracy, it is sometimes backed up by a second, more accurate test.

The second test, called *gas chromatography/mass spectrometry (GC/MS)*, is used to confirm the results of a positive screen test. The GC/MS works by providing a reading of the complete mass spectrum of an analyte as it flows through a column.

To maximize the accuracy of the GC/MS, it should be programmed to record several mass ions. For instance, a single mass ion should distinguish the target compound from sixteen others. However, three mass ions should distinguish the target compound from more than a million organic compounds. Further accuracy can be achieved by extracting, separating, derivatizing, using different ion sources, increasing resolution, and using improved packed or capillary columns.[8, 9]

To date, studies have proven that the ingestion of hempseed, whether sterilized, cooked into candy, ground into flour, or pressed into oil, causes positive urinalysis results for THC in *many* people using both the screen test and GC/MS. The THC detected in these products comes from a residue on the outside of the seed hull. After all, the highest concentrations of THC reside on the calyx that surrounds the seed.

Tests have shown that seeds that have undergone more thorough cleaning have resulted in less detectable residue and fewer positive urine tests. Daily consumption of hempseed that contains quantities of THC below 50 micrograms per gram should not be detectable in urine tests.[10] The larger hemp food producers are moving swiftly to implement more thorough cleaning processes and guaranteeing their products as THC-free (falling below the above level). Many smaller hemp food companies are standing on the principle that the problem lies with the drug labs whose tests cannot tell whether someone has smoked a joint or eaten a salad with hempseed dressing.

"Who's afraid of THC?" I ask. A few millionths of a gram of THC in a lunchbox will not affect job performance; nor will it send our kids through the gateway of drug addiction. Although this has not been verified, you'd probably have to eat several times your body weight in hempseed in a fifteen-minute period even to catch a buzz.

YOUR OPTIONS

If your freedom or livelihood is threatened because you test positive for THC after eating hempseed, consider the following options:

1. Educate the threatening party about the correlation between the ingestion of hempseed and urinalyses. Provide them with a copy of

this book; the documents cited in this chapter may be helpful. See the article from the *Journal of Analytical Toxicology* reprinted in full at the end of this chapter. See also appendix 2, "Suggested Reading." Ask that they rescind their threat and to apply this experience to hempseed eaters to follow.

2. Keep the packaging and remaining contents of the hemp foods you consume.
3. Demonstrate that hempseed is an important part of your diet. Obtain documentation supporting the unique nutritional and medicinal properties of hempseed:
    - Hempseed contains essential fatty acids (LA and LNA) in proportions ideal for our dietary needs. EFAs are essential for a healthy immune system, skin, and hair, as well as for the prevention of chronic degenerative diseases.
    - Hempseed contains gamma linolenic acid, which is absent from most common foods. GLA is beneficial for arthritis and premenstrual syndrome and is crucial to the production of prostaglandins (hormonelike chemicals that regulate nearly all cellular functions).
    - Hempseed is one of the few foods that contain all eight essential amino acids (a complete protein) in a well-balanced, easily digestible form.
    - Hempseed has the following medicinal properties: demulcent (soothes, protects, and nurtures intestinal membranes); nutritive (nourishes the body); and laxative (promotes bowel movements).
    - Hempseed is very delicious and is rapidly becoming a staple food of health-conscious people.

    Refer back to "The Healing and Nutritive Qualities of Hempseed" for more details.
4. Contact experts such as certified forensic lab analysts or hemp food experts, and ask that they back you up with expert testimony.
5. Consult with a civil rights lawyer.

6. Demonstrate that urine testing without probable cause is a violation of your fourth amendment constitutional rights (the right of the people to be secure . . . against unreasonable searches).
7. Beckon your union for help.
8. If it comes down to determining the accuracy of the test: Obtain details of every aspect of the testing process. How were the results obtained? Was a screen test performed without confirmation by a GC/MS? To how many mass ions was the analyte tested? Has the lab undergone proficiency testing? Find out the lab's record of false positives. Were there any lab mix-ups that day?

To date, after properly presenting the facts, no person has lost a job or been found to be in violation of parole when the ingestion of hempseed has resulted in a positive urinalysis for THC. But for people to undergo such suspicion and scrutiny for eating nutritious food is unacceptable.

One of the cruelest twists on this issue occurred in March 1998 when a federal judge in Los Angeles ordered cancer patient and chronic pain sufferer Todd McCormick not to use any form of marijuana, including hempseed oil, marinol, and any other product containing cannabinoid derivatives, either with or without prescription. Can you see how the phrase *cruel and unusual punishment* fits this case? For the "crime" of growing medicinal cannabis, Todd is denied the natural remedy that most helps him relieve pain and lift spirits. Not only is he forbidden from having a day without pain, but he may not even nourish his body with a food that is packed with nutrients vital to his healing.

If enough people who suffer from such injustice challenge it extensively then the institutions that require such testing, as well as institutions that provide the testing, will be forced to find methods to ensure safe workplaces that are not invasive and unconstitutional.

There is no disputing the importance of ensuring safety in the workplace, of course. Careless and irresponsible workers have the potential to cause injury to themselves, their coworkers, Mother Nature, and the public. Now that big industry insists on playing around with things such as toxic and lethal chemicals, automobiles, heavy machinery, and nuclear power, there is even greater risk.

Part of the long-term solution to keeping the workplace safe would be to use and advance the safest technologies and resources. As part of the immediate solution, we must ensure that all equipment meets safety standards and is in good repair. To minimize potential for human error, we must ensure that workers are adequately trained and skilled in their jobs.

Ensuring their competence is the easy part. Ensuring their reliability to arrive at work in peak mental and physical health, and to stay that way throughout the day, is the challenge. Instead of focusing on what comes *out* of workers' bodies as indicators of their states of mind, I believe we should be more attentive to what goes *into* their bodies.

Employers should actually be encouraging their employees to enrich their diet with hempseed. The EFA-rich seeds improve brain function and strengthen the immune system—which can result in increased mental alertness, increased stamina, and fewer sick days.

The following was originally published in the *Journal of Analytical Toxicology*, Vol. 21, July/August 1997.

A Positive THC Urinalysis from Hemp (Cannabis) Seed Oil

To the Editor:

Most varieties of hemp (i.e., non-drug *Cannabis sativa* L.) have very low levels of tetrahydrocannabinol (THC), typically less than 1.0%, although other cannabinoids may still be present in considerable amounts.[1] Even though the seed does not contain measurable amounts of any cannabinoid,[2,3] trace amounts of THC have been detected in some samples of hemp seed oil,[4] apparently from the contamination of pressed seed by adherent resin or other plant material.

We would like to report on the possibility of achieving a positive urinalysis for THC metabolite(s) after the modest consumption of commercially available hemp seed oil in *Cannabis*-naive individuals. Because hemp seed oil is an excellent source of essential fatty acids (EFAs, i.e., linoleic and linolenic acids),[5] it is sold in some stores as a dietary supplement for these and other biologically important unsaturated fatty acids. Thus, in the absence of recreational drug use, it may become necessary to consider this source as a viable explanation for cannabinoid metabolites in urine. The importance of this distinction was recently highlighted in an article that reported a positive urine test for THC metabolites after the consumption of a commercially available snack that contained hemp seeds.[6] Considering the lipophilic sequestering of THC and other cannabinoids, we were interested to know if modest consumption of hemp seed oil would result in a positive urinalysis for THC with standard laboratory methods.

In the present report, two individuals who had not used any other form of *Cannabis* consumed various amounts of commercially available hemp seed oil, which was purchased from the refrigerated section of health food stores in the Miami area. Initial urine samples, which were collected before consumption of any hemp seed oil, gave negative results by EMIT.

In a chronic experiment (experiment 1), an individual consumed approximately 10 mL/day of hemp seed oil over a period of 29 days. The oil was never heated or used in cooking, but rather applied to food just before consumption. In an acute experiment (experiment 2), another individual consumed 24 hemp seed oil capsules at one time, containing 1000 mg of oil each (24 g of oil total). Subsequent urine samples from both individuals gave positive tests for THC.

The presence of THC was determined by EMIT and verified by gas

TABLE I. EXPERIMENT 1. URINALYSES AFTER CHRONIC ADMINISTRATION OF TWO BRANDS OF HEMP SEED OIL*

Sample	Day	EMIT (ng/mL)	GC-MS (ng/mL)
1[†]	25	+[‡]	36
2[§]	27	+	72
3	29	+	87
4[ß]	32	+	66

* All urine samples were obtained from the first urination of each day.
† Sample 1 shows THC metabolite levels after the consumption of Brand A after 10 mL/day for 25 days.
‡ Positive samples exceeded the response for a 20–ng/mL calibration standard.
§ Sample 2 shows THC metabolite levels after switching to Brand B at day 27.
ß Sample 4 was obtained on day 32 after 3 days of abstinence.

chromatography—mass spectrometry (GC-MS).[7] Nearly 87 ng/mL of
Δ^9-THC-11-carboxylic acid was quantitated by GC-MS after chronic consumption of the oil (experiment 1), whereas less than 10 ng/mL was quantitated in urine samples from experiment 2.

In experiment 1, THC metabolite levels remained high after consuming 10 mL of oil per day for 25 days (Brand A). Directly following that period, 10 mL/day of another hemp seed oil (Brand B) was consumed for four additional days, followed by a three-day period of abstinence. These data are presented in Table I and show the highest levels of THC metabolite, which suggests a cumulative effect after regular consumption, along with the possibility of varying cannabinoid content in different brands of oil.

In experiment 2, the effect from an acute dose of 24 g hemp seed oil in gelatin capsules was followed over a 50-h period (Table II). In this case, THC metabolites were undetectable after 30 h, and overall metabolite levels were not as high as in experiment 1.

Low levels of THC, and probably other cannabinoids, apparently contaminate hemp seed oil as a byproduct of the extraction process. THC levels were recently reported to be 0.025% in a sample of commercial hemp seed oil and 0.375% in oil pressed from a drug variety of *Cannabis* seed,[8] presumably as the orally inactive carboxylic acid. The same study also reported no THC for oil pressed from either carefully cleaned hemp or drug-*Cannabis* seeds.

These levels are not sufficient for drug purposes, even if all THC were in an orally active form, and neither volunteer reported associated psychoactivity in the present study. However, because of the lipophilic nature of THC and other cannabinoids, bioaccumulation and subsequent excretion of metabolites can result in a positive urine test as determined by EMIT and GC-MS methodologies.

J. C. Callaway,[1] R. A. Weeks,[2] L. P. Raymon,[3]
H. C. Walls,[3] and W. L. Hearn[2]

[1]Department of Pharmaceutical Chemistry, University of Kuopio POB 1627, FIN-70211 Kuopio, Finland; [2]Dade County Medical Examiner Department, Number One Bob Hope Road, Miami, Florida 33136; and [3]Department of Pathology, Forensic Toxicology Laboratory, 12500 SW 152nd Street, Building B, Miami, Florida 33177

TABLE II. EXPERIMENT 2. URINALYSIS SUBSEQUENT TO THE ACUTE ADMINISTRATION OF 24 HEMP SEED OIL GELATIN CAPSULES*

Sample	Time of day	Elapsed time (h)	EMIT (ng/mL)	GC-MS (ng/mL)
1	07:50	2.3	+[†]	3
2	09:10	3.7	+	10
3	10:00	4.5	+	4
4	11:15	5.8	+	4
5	12:10	6.7	+	7
6	13:30	8.0	+	7
7	14:45	9.3	+/−[‡]	4
8	15:50	10.3	+/−	3
9	17:00	11.5	+	7
10	19:50	14.3	+	5
11	21:00	15.5	+/−	3
12	05:00	23.5	+/−	4
13	07:50	26.3	+	5
14	10:40	29.2	+/−	5
15	12:45	31.3	−[§]	3
16	14:30	33.0	−	2
17	17:40	36.2	−	2
18	07:55	50.4	−	3

* Each capsule contained 1000 mg oil. The entire dose (24 g) was taken at 05:00, and the first urine sample was collected at 07:50. Samples from all subsequent urinations were collected over 50 h.
† Samples exceeded the response for a 20–ng/mL calibration standard.
‡ Samples were of an intermediate value.
§ Samples were equivalent to the negative calibrator.

References

1. E. de Meijer, H. Van der Kamp, and F. Van Eeuwijk. Characterisation of Cannabis accessions with regard to cannabinoid content in relation to other plant characters. *Euphytica* 62: 187-200 (1992).

2. Botany: the unstabilized species. In *Marihuana in Science and Medicine.* M. Paris and G. G. Nahas, Eds. Raven Press, NY, 1984. pp. 3-36.

3. J. E. Viera, L. C. Abreu, and J. R. Valle. On the pharmacology of hemp seed oil. *Med. Pharmacol. Exp. (Int. J. Exp. Med.)* 16: 219-24 (1967).

4. T. Matsunaga, H. Nagatomo, I. Yamamoto, and H. Yoshimura. Identification and determination of cannabinoids in commercially available Cannabis seed. *Eisei Kagaku* 36(6): 545-47 (1990).

5. M. S. Manku. Clinical biochemistry of essential fatty acids. In *Omega-6 Essential Fatty Acids: Pathophysiology and Roles in Clinical Medicine,* D. F. Horrobin, Ed. Alan R. Liss, New York, NY, 1990. pp. 21-53.

6. Snack causes marijuana-positive drug tests. MRO Update, October 1996. p. 3.

7. R. Clouette, M. Jacob, P. Koteel, and M. Spain. Confirmation of 11-nor-Δ^9-tetrahydrocannabinol in urine as its *t*-butyldimethylsilyl derivative using GC/MS. *J. Anal. Toxicol.* 17: 1-4 (1993).

8. I Bócsa and P. Máthé. Can cannabinoids occur in hemp seed oil? *J. Hemp Assoc.* 2(2): 59 (1995).

Hempseed Farming

IT'S 1999 AND THE ONLY INDUSTRIALIZED COUNTRY that forbids the cultivation of hemp calls itself the *land of the free* . . . and prisons are the *home of the brave* cannabis farmers. Outlawing the farming of one of Earth's most important plants may be the biggest idiocy in the history of the world.

Meanwhile, farmers around the rest of the world are enjoying the opportunity to grow one of Mother Nature's best plant remedies for the ills humans have caused her.

Now Canada has joined Europe, Asia, Australia, South America, and even South Africa in the move to lift the ban on hemp cultivation and feed the growth of this potentially economically and ecologically sustainable, agricultural-based industry.

Industrial hemp is actually as legal to grow in the United States as it is in

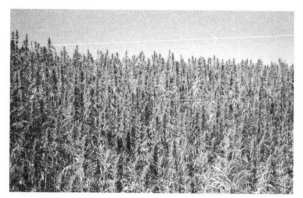

Ripe seedheads ready for harvest in a Canadian hemp field.

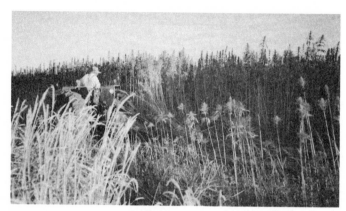

Swathing the crop.

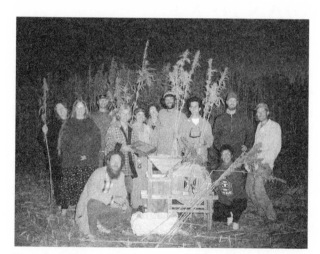

Hemp harvesters gathered around a hand-cranked winnower.

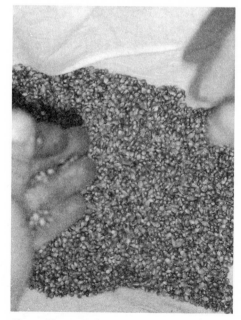

Cleaned hempseed.

Canada. So what's holding us back? Well, Canadians apply for permits to Health Canada and we apply to the Drug Enforcement Agency. On top of its paper-thin propaganda, the DEA states publicly that it never has and never will grant permits for industrial hemp cultivation. If you wish to apply anyway, then call the DEA and ask for Form 225. Clearly, we must find a way to delegate this authority to an agency that doesn't have a vested interest in prohibition.

As a matter of fact, many farmers from Kentucky and New Hampshire have filed two separate lawsuits against the DEA based on deprivation of livelihood because of the DEA's overbroad interpretation of the marijuana laws. And a recent DEA seizure of sterilized hempseed at the Canadian border poses new threats to the hemp industry.

UNITED STATES BLOCKS IMPORT OF CANADIAN HEMP

On August 9, 1999 the U.S. Drug Enforcement Agency ordered U.S. Customs at the Port of Detroit to seize a 44,000 pound shipment of sterilized hempseed valued at $25,000. The shipper, Kenex of Ontario, Canada, is a well established and respectable company that processes and distributes products made from Canadian-grown hemp. The United States market accounts for 95 percent of Kenex's business. The shipment was destined for one of the largest birdseed companies in the United States to be used as an ingredient in the company's mixes.

Without formal written notice, U.S. Customs demanded that Kenex turn over its records and recall seventeen previous shipments that date as far back as 1998 (much of which has already been consumed in food products), or face a fine in excess of $500,000. Its officers have been threatened with U.S. criminal charges and their U.S. customers have been issued with summonses to produce all records of their commercial transactions with Kenex.

This action by the DEA is clearly illegal and is inconsistent with their own policy. Sterilized hempseed is explicitly exempted from the Controlled Substance Act's definition of "marihuana":

> The term 'marihuana' means all parts of the plant Cannabis sativa (l.) . . . **BUT SHALL NOT INCLUDE** the mature stalks of such plant, fiber provided from such stalks, oil or cake made from the seeds of such plant, any other compound, manufacture, salt, derivative, mixture or preparation of such mature stalks (except the resin extracted therefrom), fiber, oil or cake or the **sterilized seed of such plant, which is incapable of germination** . . .
>
> Controlled Substances Act,
> Food and Drug Administration (1970)
> Chap. 22, Sec. 802-15

According to an October 6, 1999 press release, the DEA states, ". . . [hempseed] and products made from the seed may be contaminated with THC. Under federal law, THC is a schedule I controlled substance. Therefore, any product containing any amount of THC can only be imported into the United States by a company that is appropriately registered with DEA." This is an obvious tactical move intended to halt the hemp industry for it is almost impossible for anyone other than highly accredited medical scientists to get a Schedule I license.

Interestingly enough, the DEA's own current definition of tetrahydrocannabinol (THC) is limited to *synthetic* forms of THC, not to *organically occurring* THC such as those found in Kenex products. Industrial hempseed is also specifically highlighted in the North American Free Trade Agreement (NAFTA) as a legal U.S. import product.

Despite over sixty years of legal importation of noncleaned hempseed, the DEA instructed U.S. Customs to seize one of the cleanest loads of hempseed ever to come across the border. Today's new breed of hempseed farmers and processors have the highest standards for seed cleaning in history. The result is a product that is not only more sanitary and food grade, but contains a reduced amount of THC. The hempseed that was seized contains less than 0.001 percent THC. This percentage is fully legal under Canadian law, which allows for up to 0.3 percent THC on a whole-plant, dry-weight basis. Under the U.S. Controlled Substances Act, sterilized hempseed is not a controlled substance regardless of the THC content.

So, that leaves us with the unanswered questions of how and why the DEA would commit such a bold action that has absolutely no legal basis?

The DEA admits that it was acting on concerns over the allegations that legal hemp products could affect the outcome of urine tests. However, it is highly unlikely that any hemp product that meets Canada's strict regulations could ever affect urine tests. With urine testing in mind, Canada set a maximum limit of 10 parts per million for any hemp product. Even if someone's entire diet had a THC level of 10 ppm, the THC metabolites would remain undetected.

Fortunately, the Canadian government, some elected U.S. representatives, and several hemp industry lawyers responded quickly with pleas for the shipment to be released and to allow hempseed to be transported across the border as the law allows. The Canadian government also reminded the U.S. that this seizure action is contrary to U.S. NAFTA and World Trade Organization obligations.

According to Jean Laprise, Kenex spokesperson, the DEA notified him last week that in exchange for releasing the hempseed, Kenex must pay a seizure cost between $5,000 and $10,000 and sign a "hold harmless" agreement, which basically says the government agencies did nothing wrong and they can't be sued at a later date. Sounds like a pretty high price to pay for a shipment valued at $25,000 that was transported across the border legally in the first place.

The DEA decided to offer conditions for release only because the seed is intended for birdseed, however hempseed for human consumption would remain subject to seizure. They were unwilling to offer a guarantee that shipments of hempseed intended for either use would not be stopped at the border.

The surprisingly strong level of political support for the hemp industry forced the DEA to back down on their threats and agree to release the captive birdseed. Under this November 4, 1999 agreement with the Canadian Embassy, the DEA also instructed U. S. Customs to allow shipments of hempseed products containing trace levels of THC into the country.

This incident may have been a major setback for the hemp industry. The confidence of billion-dollar companies that the hemp industry has earned has been shaken by a single blow from a government agency acting above the law.

However, the fact that we can survive such an attack is a good sign for the hardiness and viability of hemp industries.

A happy ending is like a good dessert. May we continue to enjoy long, healthy lives with hemp!

HEMP ON THE HORIZON

In spite of bureaucratic interference, the demand in the United States for hemp products—such as clothing, fabrics, food, paper, twine, and birdseed—is shooting through the roof, but talk of domestic hemp farming is moot unless farmers show their interest in growing this crop. Let's start by organizing within the groups we currently participate in. Initiate research projects, write grants, build coalitions with Canadian hemp farmers, apply for permits—but above all keep visualizing yourself and your neighbors as organic hemp farmers. And hold true to that vision—hemp is on the horizon!

Appendix 1
Hemp Food Resource Directory

Hempseed Food Producers

Aradia's Kitchen
342 Wythe Street
Williamsburg, NY 11211
Tel: 718-388-2010
E-mail: ARADIA@acm.org
Hempseed cookies and desserts.

Boulder Hemp Company/One Brown
    Mouse
P.O. Box 1794
Nederland, CO 80466
Tel: 303-938-0195
Fax: 303-443-1869
E-mail: bhc@welcomehome.org
Web site: www.hempfoods.com
*Maker of Heavenly Hemp Foods,
including the Hemp Hotcake Mix,
Hempburger Mix, Hempizza Crust Mix,
Hemp Cookie Mix, and five flavors of
delicious Heavenly Hemp Cookies. New:
Four flavors of organic tortilla chips.*

Cannabis Candy Company
Portland, OR
Tel: 503-227-1150
Lollipops made with THC-free essential oil of cannabis flower.

Deer Garden Foods/Rejuvenative
    Foods
P.O. Box 8464
Santa Cruz, CA 95061
Tel: 800-805-7957 or 831-462-6715
Fax: 831-457-0158
Web site: www.rejuvenative.com
Producers of Hempini, the fresh, raw hulled hempseed butter, ground at low temperature.

Don Nacho's
905 Gordon Street
Victoria, BC V8W 3P9, Canada
Tel: 250-383-1959
Fax: 250-383-1959
E-mail: Omega@Bar.lover.org
Maker of the highly nutritious Omega Bar.

Dupetit Natural Products
Hauptstraße 41
63930 Richelbach, Germany
Tel: 49-9378-367
Fax: 49-9378-394
E-mail: A.DUPETIT
    @oln.comlink.apc.org
Web site: www.dupetit.de
Cannabia Beer, Hemp Tofu Pasta, and more.

Espace Nature
26, Rue des Grottes
CH-1201 Geneva, Switzerland
Tel: +41-0-22-740-4193
Fax: +41-0-22-740-4193
Cannabis tea, cakes, and pasta.

Frederick Brewing Company
4607 Wedgewood Boulevard
Frederick, MD 21703
Tel: 888-BLU-RIDG or 301-694-7899
Fax: 301-694-2971
Web site: www.hempenale.com
Producer of award-winning Hempen Ale and Hempen Gold beers.

Good Lovin'
P.O. Box 489
Paia, HI 96779
All-natural, raw, organic hempseed treats.

Greenhouse Hanf Kontor GmbH
Große Spillingsgasse 31
D-60385 Frankfurt/Main Germany
Tel: 0049-69-94592322
Fax: 0049-69-94592323
E-mail: Hanf.Kontor@t-online.de

Hempfields Natural Goods
11798 Detroit Avenue
Cleveland, OH 44107
Tel: 888-HEMP-JAVA or 216-226-0660
Fax: 216-226-2229
Web site: www.hempfields.com
Several blends of hemp coffee.

Hempfields of Hawaii
P.O. Box 752
Hilo, HI 96721
Tel: 888-HEMP-JAVA
Fax: 808-933-2113
E-mail: pakaloha@gte.net
Web site: www.hempfields.com
See above.

HempMill Specialty Coffee Roasters
4300 SanFernando Road
Glendale, CA 91204
Tel: 877-BREW-HEMP or 818-547-9291
Fax: 818-548-4538
Web site: www. hempmill.com
Health Conscious Coffee, Presidential Blends, HempMill House Blends, Flavored Hemp Bean, certified organic, shade-grown blends.

HempNut, Incorporated
P.O. Box 1368
Santa Rosa, CA 95402-1368
Tel: 707-571-1330
Fax: 707-545-7116
E-mail: info@TheHempNut.com
Web site: www.TheHempNut.com
Makers of the HempNut family of foods as well as HempRella and Hempeh Burgers.

Hempola
3405 American Drive
Ste. 5
Mississauga, ON
L4V 1T6 Canada
Tel: 800-240-9215 or 905-678-1066
Fax: 905-678-6036
Web site: www.hempola.com
Hemp oil, salad dressing, soaps, and related products.

Hempstead, Inc.
2060 Placentia
Costa Mesa, CA 92627
Tel: 714-650-8325
Fax: 714-650-5853
Web site: www.hempstead.com
Importer of nonsterilized hempseed oil.

Hemp Essentials
Box 151
Cazadero, CA 95421
Tel: 707-847-3642
Food and body care products. Owner Carol Miller is coauthor of The Hemp Seed Cookbook.

Hemp Network
P.O. Box 11008
Portland, OR 97211
Tel: 503-284-2589
E-mail: hempnetwork@hempseed.com
Web site: www.hempnetwork.com
Producers of I.P. Freedom! Bars.

Hemp Wine America
60 Grand Boulevard
Binghamton, NY 13905
Tel: 888-520-9463
Fax: 607-766-0222
Web site: www.hempwine.com
Working with established wineries in the Finger Lakes, New York, region to produce Nirvana Homebrews' Hemp Wine.

Hempzels/No Problem, Inc.
P.O. Box 13
New Holland, PA 17557
Tel: 800-USE-HEMP or 717-354-9315
Fax: 717-354-2335
E-mail: iriemon@redrose.net
Maker of gourmet hand-rolled, hearth-baked hemp pretzels.

Humboldt Brewing Company
856 10th Street
Arcata, CA 95521
Tel: 707-826-1734
Fax: 707-826-2045
Web site: www.humbrew.com
Microbrewer of Humboldt Hemp Ale, distributed throughout California.

Humboldt Hemp Foods
P.O. Box 99
Whitehorne, CA 95589
Tel: 707-986-7759
Fax: 707-986-7759
Hemp flour and cake mixes; "Sumatra Sativa" Organic Hempseed Coffee; Oh Mega organic blue corn/hulled hempseed chips.

Kenex, Ltd.
R.R. #1
Pain Court
Ontario, N0P 120
Tel: 519-351-9922
Fax: 519-352-6667
E-mail: Kenex@kent.net
Web site: www.kenex.org
Producers, processors, and suppliers of certified, O.E.C.D. approved hempseed, grain hemp for processing, oil, seed meal, hulled hempseed, and fiber products.

LaChanvrière de l'Aube
10 200 Bar-sur-Aube, France
Tel: 33-0-3-2592-3192
Fax: 33-0-3-2527-3548
Web site: www.marisy.fr/chanvriere
Hemp oil, plus much more.

Limestone Brewing Company
900 West Maxwell Street
Lexington, KY 40508
Tel: 606-252-6004
Fax: 606-259-2736
Brewer of Kentucky Hemp Beer.

Mr. Spinners
1003 Royal Oak Avenue
New Westminister, BC, V3M 1K3, Canada
Tel: 604-522-9480
E-mail: italspin@hotmail.com
Organic hemp functional foods.

Natur Art
Gimborner Str. 98
51709 Marienheide, Germany
Tel: +49-2264-286990
Fax: +49-2264-28418
E-mail: ifhemp@t-online.de
Bulk purchase: hempseed, flour, hulled hempseed, oil, muesli, spread, pasta, chocolate, beer, applejuice, canna ice tea, and Canalade.

New Earth
4652 Clark
Montreal, QB, Canada
Tel: 514-282-6579
Fax: 514-282-4166
Maker of the Boom Bar; supplier of seeds.

New Earth Ltd.
P.O. Box 204
Barnet, London EN5 1EP, England
Tel: 010-44-0-378-559-242
Web site: www.hemp.co.uk
Producer of 9-Bar and other hemp foods; supplier of organic hempseed.

Northern Lights Hemp Company
Box 591
Tofino, BC, V0R 2Z0, Canada
Tel: 800-880-3699 or 250-725-4288
Fax: 250-725-4288
E-mail: mama@island.net
Web site: www.island.net/~mama
Maker of Mama Indica's Hemp Seed Treats and roasted hempseed.

Omega Nutrition U.S.A., Inc.
6515 Aldrich Road
Bellingham, WA 98226
Tel: 800-661-3529
Fax: 800-661-3529
E-mail: omega@istar.ca
Web site: www.omegaflo.com
Producer of certified organic, fresh-pressed hempseed oil. Fresh-pressed means the seeds are dated and only the freshest are pressed using the Omegaflo process.

Omega Nutrition Canada, Inc.
1924 Franklin Street
Vancouver, BC V5L 1R2, Canada
See Omega Nutrition USA, Inc.

Original Sources
Box 7137
Boulder, CO 80306
Tel: 970-225-8356 or 303-237-3579
Domestically produced hempseed oil, HempScream, cookies, flour, and much more. Conducts R&D with hemp foods and biodiesel fuel.

Pacific Hemp Associates
P.O. Box 1084
Aptos, CA 95001
Tel: 408-688-8706
Fax: 408-688-8711
E-mail: info@pacifichemp.com
Web site: www.pacifichemp.com
Producer of nonsterilized organic hempseed oil, seed cake, and flour.

Rella Good Cheese Company
P.O. Box 5020
Santa Rosa, CA 95402-5020
Tel: 707-527-5711
Fax: 707-545-7116
E-mail: info@rella.com
Web site: www.rella.com
Producer of HempRella and Hempeh Burgers.

Sativa's Kitchen
5243 Highway 9
Felton, CA 95018
Tel: 408-438-4510
Fax: 408-439-3251
E-mail: sativa@pacifichemp.com
Web site: www.pacific.com/sativa
Maker of Hempseed Oil Pesto and desserts.

Spectrum Naturals
133 Copeland Street
Petaluma, CA 94952
Tel: 800-995-2705
Fax: 707-765-1026
E-mail: spectrumnaturals@netdex.com
Web site: www.spectrumnaturals.com
Producer of cold-pressed hempseed oil.

Star Trade
Box 184 CH-8184
Bachenbülach, Switzerland
Tel: +41-1-862-2057
Fax: +41-1-862-2040
E-mail: info@swisscannabis.com
Web site: www.swisscannabis.com
Maker of Swiss Cannabis Pastilles,

throat lozenges made with essential oil of cannabis blossoms.

Teco Finance Export
24 Rue Violet
75015 Paris, France
Tel: 331-45-78-92-91
Fax: 331-45-77-00-69
Producer and exporter of hempseed oil.

Valchanvre Sarl
Ferme l'Oasis, CH-1907
Saxon, Switzerland
Fax: 41-27-744-39-28
E-mail: valchanvre@omedia.ch
Web site: www.omedia.ch/silicon/
    valchanvre
Hemp oil, perfumes, cosmetics.

Vermont Hemp Co./Green Horizons
P.O. Box 5233
Burlington, VT 05402
Tel: 802-878-9089
E-mail: vthempco@hempseed.com
Web site: www.freeyellow.com/
    members/javahemp
Huge line of hemp foods for humans (and dogs).

Willie's Hemp Soda Co.
454 Las Gallinas Avenue #207
San Rafael, CA 94903
Tel: 877-TRY-HEMP or 415-479-6250
Fax: 415-479-7350
E-mail: willizing@willieshemp.com
Web site: www. wllieshemp.com
Manufacturer of nautral hemp sodas and other specialty beverages.

Zima Foods
P.O. Box 5982, Station B
Victoria, BC, V8R 6S8, Canada
Tel: 250-381-7333
Fax: 250-388-4873
E-mail:zima@ampsc.com
Web site: www.cinevision.com/zima/
    z.html
*All-natural raw organic hempseed
delicacies and catering.*

Restaurants Serving Hemp Food

Blue Sun Café
True Nature Foods
13070 Highway 9
Boulder Creek, CA 95006
Tel: 408-308-2105
*Café and catering service serving up a
gargantuan hemp feast.*

The Galaxy Global Eatery
15 Irving Place
New York, NY 10003
Tel: 212-777-3631
Fax: 212-777-3224
E-mail: galstar@aol.com
Web site: www.galaxyglobaleatery.com
*Serving fresh and inventive foods
made with hemp; also sells its own
brand of hempseed oil and coffee.*

White Light Diner
114 Bridge St.
Frankfort, KY 40601
Tel: 502-227-4889
*Serves hempseed baked goods and beef
from cows fed with hempseed.*

Distributors of Hemp Food Products: Wholesale

Impex International Corporation
Bonita Springs, FL 34135
*U.S. distributor of Swiss Canabis
Pastilles.*

The Hemp Club THC, Inc.
3418 A Park Avenue
Montreal, QC, H2X 2H5, Canada
Tel: 514-845-4993
Fax: 514-845-4687
E-mail: thehempclubthc@hotmail.com
*Canadian distributor of Swiss Can-
nabis Pastilles.*

Mountain People's Warehouse
12745 Earhart Avenue
Auburn, CA 95602
Tel: 800-679-8735
Fax: 530-889-1182
*(Hemp) Rella Good Cheese, Hempeh
Burgers, Merry Hempsters Lip Balm,
Sue's Amazing Lip Stuff.*

Mountain People's Northwest
P.O. Box 81106
Seattle, WA 98106-1106
Tel: 800-336-8872 outside Washington,
    or 800-762-0211 in-state
Fax: 800-210-0104
See entry above.

Suppliers of Seeds and Oil: Wholesale

Atlas Corporation
4676 Admiralty Way, Ste. 410
Marina del Rey, CA 90292-6695
Tel: 310-335-2028
Fax: 310-306-0173
E-mail: erik@atlascor.com

Australian Hemp Products
P.O. Box 23
Newlambton, NSW
Newcastle, Australia 2305
Tel: +61-249-55-6666
Fax: +61-249-55-6655
E-mail: austhemp@hunterlink.net.au

BioHemp Ltd.
P.O. Box 21590 Little Italy Post Office
Vancouver, BC, V5N 5T5, Canada
E-mail: jfreeman@ssm.net
Marketers of Canadian certified organic hempseed and oil.

Canadian Hemp Corporation
Sidney, B.C.
Tel: 250-656-7233
Fax: 250-656-8860
E-mail: hempcorp@home.com
Offers Canadian-grown hempseed oil and seed cake.

Finola
P.O. Box 236
FIN-70100 KUOPIO, Finland
Web site: www.finola.com
Producers of unfiltered oil cold-pressed from a high latitude strain called FIN-314, grown in Finland. Nitrogen sealed in dark glass bottles.

Global Hemp
307 E. Melbourne Ave.
Peoria, IL 61603
Tel: 309-685-3591
E-mail: info@globalhemp.com
Web site: www. globalhemp.com

Green Lands Ecological Hemp Products
P.O. Box 1651
1000 BR Amsterdam, Netherlands
Tel: 31-020-625-1100
Fax: 31-020-422-1125
Producer and wholesaler of hempseed oil, food and seed products, and clothes.

Hempseed Organics Ltd.
P.O. Box 11797
London N15 6NQ, England
Tel: 0170-833-3178
Fax: 0170-833-3178
E-mail: hempseed@gn.apc.org
Supplier of organic hempseed.

Herbal Products and Development
P.O. Box 1084
Aptos, CA 95001
Tel: 408-688-8706
Fax: 408-688-8711
Supplier of nonsterilized hempseed oil; formulators of Supreme 7 oil blend.

IF-Gebr. Bernhardt
Gimborner Str. 96 B-98
51709 Marienheide, Germany
Tel: +49-2264-28418
Fax: +49-2264-28418
Hempseed oil, seeds, flour, and much more.

La Chanvrière de l'Aube
See entry under Hempseed Farming.

The Ohio Hempery
7002 State Route 329
Guysville, OH 45735
Tel: 800-BUY-HEMP
Fax: 614-662-6446
E-mail: hempery@hempery.com
Web site: www.hempery.com
Suppliers of sterilized seed, hempseed oil, hempseed cake, cosmetic-grade oil, and hemp by-products.

Animal Feed Suppliers

The Ohio Hempery
7002 State Route 329
Guysville, OH 45735
Tel: 800-BUY-HEMP
Fax: 614-662-6446
E-mail: hempery@hempery.com
Web site: www.hempery.com
Hempseed meal.

Pacific Hemp
See entry under Hempseed Food Producers.

Hempseed Farming

Hempco/Shazam Farms
2720 Way's Mills Road
Ayer's Cliff, Quebec
J0B 1C0, Canada
Tel: 819-838-5832
Fax: 819-838-5218
E-mail: hempco@interlinx.qc.ca
Producers of certified organic hempseed and fiber.

Island Hemp Co.
RR2 Point Pleasant
Murray River, P.E.I.
C0A 1W0, Canada
E-mail: islandhemp@pei.sympatico.ca
Farming, processing, and sales of hempseed, fiber, pulp, and hurd.

La Chanvrière de l'Aube
Rue du Général de Gaulle
F-10 200 Bar sur Aube, France
Tel: +33 (0)3-25923192
fax: +33 (0)3-25273548
E-mail: www.canvre.com
Producers and suppliers of hempseed oil and fiber products.

Hemp Food Consulting and Other Services

Australian Hemp
    Resource and Manufacture
P.O. Box 426
Ashgrove, QLD
Australia 4060
Tel: 61-7-3366-0889
Fax: 61-7-3366-0890
Research and brokering of hemp products and resources, expanding into hemp foods.

Hungry Bear Hemp Foods
P.O. Box 12175
Eugene, OR 97440-4375
E-mail: eathemp@efn.org
Web site: www.efn.org/~eathemp/
    hbhempfood.html
Author of this book. I consult with
producers, restaurants, retailers; assist in product creation and marketing; give workshops and lectures.

J. C. Callaway, Ph.D.
Department of Pharmaceutical
    Chemistry
University of Kuopio
P.O. Box 1627
FIN-70211 KUOPIO, Finland
Tel: +358-17-163-601
Fax: +358-17-162-456
Web site: www. finola.com
Consultant specializing in cannabis biochemistry, breeding, and nutrition.

Transglobal Hemp Products Corporation
P.O. Box 8748
Victoria, BC, V8W 3S3, Canada
Tel: 250-384-4873
Fax: 250-388-4873
Industry developer for Vancouver Island.

Richard Rose
(See entries for HempNut, Incorpo-
    rated, and Rella Good Cheese
    Company)
Hempseed food product and process development and marketing; nineteen years' full-time experience.

Business Associations

Australian Hemp Industries Association
P.O. Box 236
Newlambton, Newcastle,
NSW, Australia 2305
Tel: +61-249-556666
Fax: +61-249-556655
E-mail: austhemp@hurterlink.net.au

Canadian Hemp Growers Association
5811 156th St.
Surrey, BC, V3S 8E7
Canada
Tel: 604-506-2352
U.S. Tel/Fax: 360-945-0295
E-mail: delta3@whidbey.com
Non-profit resource providing member networking, education, and information.

Canadian Industrial Hemp Council
P.O. Box 36035
Halifax, NS
B3J 3S9, Canada
Tel: 902-477-6686
Fax: 902-477-1017
E-mail: cihc@hotmail.com
Farmers, manufacturers, wholesalers, retailers, and students who assist in the development of the regulatory framework for the legalization of industrial hemp in Canada.

Hemp Food Association
P.O. Box 1368
Santa Rosa, CA 95402-1368
Tel: 707-571-1330
Fax: 707-545-7116
E-mail: Info@hempfood.com
Web site: www.hempfood.com

Hemp Food Industries Association
P.O. Box 204
Barnet, London EN5 1EP, England
To promote and support manufacturers, wholesalers, retailers, and end-users of hemp food products as well as to gain awareness of other legal uses of the hemp plant.

HIA—Hemp Industries Association
P.O. Box 1080
Occidental, CA 95465
Tel: 707-874-3648
Fax: 707-874-1104
E-mail: Info@thehia.org
Web site: www.thehia.org

Hemp Industries Marketing Board of
    New Zealand, Ltd.
P.O. Box 11-015
Wellington, New Zealand
Tel: 64-4-382-8607
Fax: 64-4-385-4855
Import, manufacture, export, brokerage.

IHA—International Hemp Association
Postbus 75007
1070 AA Amsterdam, Netherlands
Tel: 31-20-618-8758
E-mail: Iha@euronet.nl
Nonprofit organization dedicated to the advancement of the cannabis plant through the dissemination of information. Publishes the biennial Journal of IHA.

Kentucky Hemp Growers Cooperative
      Association, Inc.
P.O. Box 8395
Lexington, KY 40533
Tel: 606-252-8954
E-mail: WdavidS100@aol.com
Incorporated in 1942, this association serves to establish and promote market equity among industrial hemp suppliers, processors, and manufacturers.

New Zealand Hemp Industries
      Association, Inc.
P.O. Box 38 392
Howick, Auckland, New Zealand
Tel: +64-9-273-2541
Fax: +64-9-273-7396
E-mail: nzhemp@es.co.nz
A non-profit organization supporting the local hemp industry by facilitating the exchange of information and expertise, while lobbying the New Zealand government.

NAIHC—North American Industrial
      Hemp Council
P.O. Box 259329
Madison, WI 53725-9329
Tel: 608-224-5135
Fax: 608-224-5110
E-mail: sholtea@wheel.datcp.state.wi.us
Web site: www.naihc.com

Swiss Hemp Co-Ordination
Tel: +41-01-450-6185
Fax: +41-01-450-6186
E-mail: reusser@dial.eunet.ch
Organization of Swiss hemp businesses.

Useful Hemp Food-Crafting Supplies

Real Goods
555 Leslie Street
Ukiah, CA 95482-5507
Tel: 800-762-7325
Fax: 707-468-0301
Supplier of the Corona flour mill, kitchen goods, and many hemp products.

Retsel Corporation
Box 47
McCammon, Idaho 83250
Tel: 800-854-8862
Fax: 208-254-3325
Manufacturers of hand-cranked and electric flour mills suitable for families, restaurants, and small food producers.

Pak-Sel
7205 S.E. Johnson Creek Rd.
Portland, OR 97206
Tel: 800-635-2247
Fax: 503-771-9413
Distributor of Champion, Omega, and Phoenix juicers. Manufacturers of cellulose (plant fiber) bags.

APPENDIX 1

Appendix 2
Suggested Reading

Bennett, Chris, Lynn Osburn, and Judy Osburn. *Green Gold the Tree of Life: Marijuana in Magic and Religion.* Frazier Park, Calif.: Access Unlimited, 1995.

Bócsa, Iván, and Michael Karus. *The Cultivation of Hemp.* Sebastopol, Calif.: Hemptech, 1998. *Botany, cultivation, and harvesting*

Brown, Edward Espe. *The Tassajara Bread Book.* Boulder, Colo.: Shambhala, 1995. *A highly recommended book on the fine craft of whole grain bread making.*

Callaway, J.C., Weeks, R.A., Raymon, L.P., Walls, H.C., and Hearn, W.L. "A Positive THC Urinalysis from Hemp (Cannabis) Seed Oil." *Journal of Analytical Toxicology* 21, no. 4 (1997).

Commins, John. "Kids' Sweet Snack Flunks Lab's Drug Test." *Nashville Banner*, 27 August 1996.

Conrad, Chris. *Hemp for Health.* Rochester, Vt.: Healing Arts Press, 1997.

———. *Hemp: Lifeline to the Future.* Los Angeles: Creative Xpressions, 1994.

Erasmus, Udo. *Fats That Heal, Fats That Kill.* Burnaby, B.C.: Alive Books, 1996. *Authoritative and easy-to-understand guide to dietary* fats. Many references to hempseed oil as a good source of EFAs.

Flowers, Tom. *Marijuana Herbal Cookbook*. Oakland, Calif.: Flowers Publishing, 1995.

Gaskin, Stephen. *Cannabis Spirituality*. New York: High Times Books, 1996.

Gottlieb, Adam. *The Art and Science of Cooking with Cannabis*. Berkeley, Calif.: Ronin Publishing, 1993.

Harrison, Lewis. *Making Fats & Oils Work for You*. Garden City, N.Y.: Avery Publishing Group, 1990. *A consumer's guide that is easier to understand, but less authoritative, than* Fats That Heal, Fats That Kill.

Herer, Jack. *The Emperor Wears No Clothes*. Van Nuys, Calif.: AH HA Publishing, 1998. *This is the eleventh edition of the book that helped launch the movement, and it takes a giant leap in the quality of its appearance and of its content.*

Jones, Kenneth. *Nutritional and Medicinal Guide to Hemp Seed*. Gibsons, B.C.: Rainforest Botanical Laboratory, 1995.

Larson, Gero, Petra Pless, and John Roulac. *Hemp Foods and Oils for Health*. Sebastopol, Calif.: Hemptech, 1991.

M. R. P. "'Seedy Sweetie' Snack Bars Blamed for THC-Positive Test." *Drug Detection Report*, 21 October 1996.

Miller, Carol, and Don Wirtshafter. *The Hemp Seed Cookbook*. Athens, Ohio: Hempery, 1994. *A 21-page booklet on basic whole-seed hemp food-crafting.*

Mosley, Joe. "'Seedy' Market Blossoms." *The Register Guard* (Eugene, Oreg.), 30 August 1996.

Potter, Beverly, and Dan Joy. *The Healing Magic of Cannabis*. Berkeley, Calif.: Ronin Publishing, 1998.

Rathbun, Mary, and Dennis Peron. *Brownie Mary's Marijuana Cookbook*. San Francisco: Trail of Smoke Publishing, 1996.

Robertson, Laurel, and Carol Flinders. *The Laurel's Kitchen Bread Book*. New York: Random House, 1985. *A highly recommended book on the fine craft of whole grain bread making.*

Robertson, Laurel, Brian Ruppenthal, and Carol Flinders. *The New Laurel's Kitchen—A Handbook for Vegetarian Cookery and Nutrition*. Berkeley, Calif.: Ten Speed Press, 1986.

Robinson, Rowan. *The Great Book of Hemp*. Rochester, Vt.: Park Street Press, 1996.

Rosenthal, Ed (ed.). *Hemp Today*. Oakland, Calif.: Quick American Archives, 1994.

Roulac, John W. *Hemp Horizons*. White River Junction, Vt.: Chelsea Green, 1997.

Sloman, Larry. *Reefer Madness*. Indianapolis, N.Y.: Bobbs-Merrill, 1979.

Starks, Michael. *Marijuana Chemistry*. Berkeley, Calif.: Ronin Publishing, 1990.

Notes

Hempseed Overview

1. Iván Bócsa, and Michael Karus, *The Cultivation of Hemp* (Sebastopol, Calif.: Hemptech, 1998), 19.
2. Claudius Galen, *De Facultatibus Alimentorum*, 100.49, cited in Chris Conrad, *Hemp: Lifeline to the Future* (Los Angeles: Creative Expressions, 1994), 11-12.
3. Ernest Abel, *Marijuana, The First Twelve Thousand Years* (New York: Plenum Press, 1980), cited in Kenneth Jones, *Nutritional and Medicinal Guide to Hemp Seed* (Gibson, B.C.: Rainforest Botanical Laboratory, 1995), 24-25 and 32-35.
4. Kenneth Jones, *Nutritional and Medicinal Guide to Hempseed* (Gibson, B.C.: Rainforest Botanical Laboratory, 1995), 21.
5. Ibid.
6. J. M. Watt, and M. G. Breyer-Brandwijk, *The Medicinal & Poisonous Plants of Southern Africa* (Edinburgh: E & S Livingtone, 1932), cited in Conrad, 12.

The Healing and Nutritive Qualities of Hempseed

1. Lynn Osburn, "Hemp Seed: The Most Nutritionally Complete Food Source In the World, Part One," *Hemp Line Journal* 1 (July–August 1992): 14-15.
2. Chris Conrad, *Hemp: Lifeline to the Future* (Los Angeles: Creative Expressions, 1994), 141.
3. Udo Erasmus, *Fats That Heal, Fats That Kill* (Burnaby, B.C.: Alive Books, 1996), 270-71.
4. From studies of evening primrose oil by Dr. David Horrobin, cited in Erasmus, 272.
5. Erasmus, 47, 48.
6. Herbert L. Meltzer, *The Chemistry of Human Behavior* (Chicago: Nelson-Hall, 1979), 21.
7. J. Singh, R. Hamid, and B. S. Reddy, "Dietary Fat and Colon Cancer: Modulating Effect of Types and Amount of Dietary Fat on ras-p21 Function during Promotion and Progression Stages of Colon Cancer," *Cancer Research* 57 (1997), 253-58, cited in Artemis P. Simopoulos, M.D., *The Omega Plan* (New York: HarperCollins, 1988), 25.
8. Erasmus, 51.
9. Conrad, 11.
10. Ibid.
11. D. Bensky, and A. Gamble, *Chinese Herbal Medicine: Materia Medica* (Seattle: Eastland Press, 1993), 120, cited in Jones, 8-9.
12. Michael Tierra, *Planetary Herbology* (Santa Fe: Lotus Press, 1988), 173.
13. F. Porter Smith, *Chinese Materia Medica, Vegetable Kingdom* (Taipei, Taiwan: KuT'ing Book House, 1969), 90-91, cited in Jones, 12.
14. Horrobin, cited in Erasmus, 272.
15. Ibid.
16. Kun-Ying Yen, *The Illustrated Chinese Materia Medica Crude and Prepared* (Taipei, Taiwan: SMC Publishing, Inc., 1992), 164, cited in Jones, 9.
17. Ibid, 317-18.
18. Horrobin, cited in Erasmus, 272.
19. Porter, cited in Jones, 12.
20. Yen 323-24, cited in Jones, 9.
21. Jones, 7-19.
22. Singh, Hamid, and Reddy, cited in Simopoulous, 25.
23. Ibid.
24. Ibid.
25. Norman Goudry, trans. "Da Ma (Hemp, Marijuana—*Cannabis sativa*)" *Translations from the Ben Cao Gang Mu* (Madeira Park, B.C., 1995) cited in Jones 15-18.
26. Sing, Hamid, and Reddy, cited in Simopuolos, 25.
27. Ibid.

Friendly Fungus

1. Paul Stamets, *Growing Gourmet and Medicinal Mushrooms* (Olympia, Wash.: Mycomedia Production, 1993), 6.

2. Ibid., 10.
3. David W. Fischer, and Alan E. Bessette, *Edible Wild Mushrooms of North America* (Austin, Tex.: University of Texas Press, 1992), 4–5.

Hempseed Underground
1. Barbara Grunes, and Ann Elise Hunt, *Roots: The Underground Cookbook* (Chicago, Ill.: Chicago Review Press, 1993), 6.

Food for Feathers, Fins, and Four Legs
1. Dave Baker, "It's Not Pot: White Light Diner Serves Hemp Burgers and Hemp Seed Muffins," *The State Journal* (Frankfort, Ky.), 3 June 1998, front page.
2. Janet Patton, "Hemp: From Seed to Feed," *Lexington* (Ky.) *Herald-Leader*, 27 May 1998, business section.
3. Ibid.
4. Baker, *The State Journal*, 3 June 1998.
5. Erasmus, 43.
6. Janet Patton, "KSU Researchers Investigating Hemp as Food for Catfish," *Lexington* (Ky.) *Herald-Leader*, 27 May 1998, business section.
7. Jack Herer, *The Emperor Wears No Clothes* (Van Nuys, Calif.: AH HA Publishing, 1998), 10, 53.

Free to Pee THC
1. John Commins, "Kids' Sweet Snack Flunks Lab's Drug Test," *Nashville Banner* (Nashville, Tenn.), 27 August 1996.
2. Joe Mosley, "'Seedy' Market Blossoms," *The Register Guard* (Eugene, Oreg.), 30 August 1996, 1B, 3B.
3. M.R.P., "'Seedy Sweetie' Snack Bars Blamed for THC-Positive Test," *Drug Detection Report* (PaceCom, Inc.), 21 October 1996.
4. P. Armentano and A. St. Pierre, NORML Foundation, "Jury Overturns Court-Martial After Hearing Marine Consumed Legal Hemp Oil," HIA bulletin, 8 May 1998.
5. J. C. Callaway, R. A. Weeks, L. P. Raymon, H. C. Walls, and W. L. Hearn, "A Positive THC Urinalysis from Hemp (Cannabis) Seed Oil," *Journal of Analytical Toxicology*, 21, no. 4: letter to the editor.
6. M. R. P. , *Drug Detection Report.*
7. Dale G. Deutsch, ed., *Analytical Aspects of Drug Testing* (New York: John Wiley & Sons, 1989), 273–91.
8. Ibid.
9. Joseph Chamberlain, *The Analysis of Drugs in Biological Fluids*, 2nd ed. (New York: CRS Press, 1995), 119.
10. Swiss Academy of Sciences.

INDEX

INDEX

● ● ●

184

Glenview Public Library
1930 Glenview Road
Glenview, Illinois

3 1170 00533 9134